Here are specific and startling scientific facts about the healing power of foods . . .

- An **APPLE** a day actually can keep the doctor away because "the king of fruits" contains a smorgasbord of nutrients and phytochemicals including soluble fiber, boron, iron, vitamin B_2 and potassium. These are known to fight cancer and infection, lower cholesterol, balance blood sugar, strengthen bones and even relieve menopausal symptoms.

- **FISH** contains a fatty acid called "omega-3" which can decrease the risk of coronary artery disease by up to 40%. In addition, eating fish can help to control diabetes, reduce arthritis symptoms and cholesterol, and aid in the battle against eczema and psoriasis.

- Revered for centuries as a natural medicine, the "stinking rose" or **GARLIC** is now widely regarded as a serious cancer-fighter even by the National Cancer Institute. It contains over 30 anti-carcinogenic substances, including vitamins C and B_6, potassium, selenium, phosphorus, fluorine, bioflavonoids and allicin. Magical garlic will also diminish aging, reduce cholesterol, relieve arthritis, aid in digestion and fight a myriad of respiratory problems.

- Plain lowfat **YOGURT** is an excellent source of B_{12}, calcium, magnesium and potassium and its "live" probiotic cultures can boost the immune system, prevent diarrhea and ward off yeast infections.

FOODS TO HEAL BY

BARRY FOX, Ph.D.

Foreword by Arnold Fox, M.D.

A LYNN SONBERG BOOK

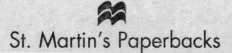

St. Martin's Paperbacks

To my wife, Nadine.

Published by arrangement with:
Lynn Sonberg Book Associates
10 West 86 Street
New York, NY 10024

FOODS TO HEAL BY

ISBN: 0-312-95987-7

Printed in the United States of America

St. Martin's Paperbacks edition/November 1996

10 9 8 7 6 5 4 3 2 1

Important Note to Readers

Contents

Foreword

by Arnold Fox, M.D.

As an internist and cardiologist who has treated countless patients, I like to think of good nutrition and foods as my "first choice" medicine, when appropriate. And it is often appropriate. I've seen many patients struggling with arthritis—and with the side effects of arthritis medications—who benefited tremendously from simple changes in diet. Many diabetics have been able to slowly cut back on their insulin, and eventually get off it all together. Heart patients have avoided seemingly inevitable heart attacks and surgery thanks to a combination of good nutrition, exercise, and stress reduction. Good nutrition has even helped cancer patients to enjoy an improved sense of well-being (which is an important medicine in and of itself). And who knows how many people have never had these diseases at all, thanks in large part to the foods they ate?

If I could redesign the typical doctor's "little black bag," I would fill it with lots of fresh fruits and vegetables, with whole grains and legumes, with lean meats and dairy products. There would be medicines for people with serious or acute illnesses, of course, but we doctors would focus on avoiding illness. How? In large part by using healthful foods to strengthen our patients' immune systems, by filling their bodies with the vitamins, minerals, phytochemicals, and other components of foods that are proven disease-fighters.

Many people have asked me which foods are best, and what healthful effects they have. Fortunately, they can now find the answers to all of their food-as-medicine questions in *Foods to Heal By,* a superb compilation of the healing effects of foods. This is exactly the kind of book my patients ask me for. It's up-to-date, detailed yet easy to read, and stuffed with well-researched information. And you choose how to use this book. You can take a quick look at the healing properties of the foods, or you can delve into the scientific studies often discussed below the brief overview of healing properties. Or you can do both. It's up to you.

I have to admit to being a little biased about this book. After all, it was written by my son Barry, the little baby I used to bounce on my knee, the boy who loved playing baseball, and the man with whom I've written eight books. Now he's beautifully wed style and substance to produce an in-depth encyclopedia of the healing effects of foods. Foods are indeed natural healers. And *Foods to Heal By* is a wonderful guide to the marvelous, medicinal world of foods.

Introduction

The healing powers of foods have been known since at least the dawn of recorded history. The ancient Egyptians, Greeks, Romans, Hebrews, and others used foods to treat a variety of ailments, from hangovers to heart disease. But as powerful new antibiotics and other new medicines burst onto the medical scene in the first half of the twentieth century, the medicinal qualities of foods were forgotten by many physicians and scientists. Still, even though the medical establishment focused on drugs, some doctors and researchers continued studying the benefits of foods and the various substances in foods. Many patients and other people, too, continued to rely on foods to help prevent or relieve the symptoms of many diseases.

Then, in the 1970s, the startling results of decades of methodical research forced the medical establishment to begin rethinking its position. Why did populations eating high-fat diets tend to suffer from greater rates of heart disease and cancer? Why did people's diseases change as they moved from country to country and adopted new diets? Was there more to food than filling the belly and providing some nutrients? Could foods somehow prevent or treat diseases?

The answer is a resounding yes! Even the most conservative and drug-oriented of health organizations now agree that food is a powerful medicine. The Food & Nutrition Board, the organization which sets the RDAs (Recommended Dietary Allowances), has stated that: *"There are clear-cut ways for reducing your risk of disease by modifying your diet."* A co-author of the Board's 1992 nine-point dietary plan added: *"Without sacrificing favorite foods, but by modifying and balancing the types of foods eaten, diet could substantially reduce the number of Americans who die prematurely from heart disease, cancer and other chronic diseases."*

Many other prominent health organizations have spoken up in favor of using food as medicine. As the American Dietetic Association has noted: *"The philosophy that food can be health promoting beyond its nutritional value is gaining acceptance within the public arena and among the scientific community as mounting research links diet/food components to disease prevention and treatment."*

Many consumers believe in the healing powers of nutrients and other substances in food, spending more than $4 billion in 1994 on vitamins, minerals, herbs, and other nutritional supplements. Supplements by themselves, however, are not as good as whole foods. Although most of us are familiar with beta-carotene, few of us realize that it is only one of hundreds of different carotenes in vegetables and fruits. There are many other medicinal substances in foods, including bioflavonoids, coumarins, indoles, isoflavones, and more that have not been put into supplements, with many more food substances yet to be identified and understood. It's clear that food is much more than the sum of its vitamins and minerals. Someday, perhaps, we'll be able to duplicate food in pill form. Until then, the best bet is to "medicate" ourselves with the well-known and the still-mysterious ingredients in foods that energize our immune systems, keep our brains sharp, ward off cancer, keep the coronary arteries wide open, and otherwise help to keep us healthy and happy.

HOW THIS BOOK WILL HELP YOU

You can use *Foods to Heal By* as a "quick look" reference to individual foods, nutrients, and diseases, or as a detailed guide to the marvelous healing powers of foods.

Chapter 1 presents an overview of the medicinal power of food. Over twenty-five of the most common diseases and conditions are briefly described, and some of the foods that help to control or prevent them are presented. If you read only this chapter, you will learn enough to make basic dietary changes that will help to set you on the road to health and longevity.

But if you're interested in learning more about the sub-stances in foods that energize the immune system, retard ag-ing, and help to prevent or cure numerous diseases, continue reading. Chapters 2, 3, and 4 delve into the healing powers of vitamins and minerals, plus the many other healing substances (phytochemicals) in foods that fight disease and encourage health.

Finally, Chapter 5 carefully examines close to one hundred common foods, from alfalfa sprouts to yogurt. Each of the food's healing powers is described, and, when appropriate, supporting scientific studies are described. Tips for including the foods in your diet and a detailed breakdown of what each food contains are also presented. Armed with the information in this chapter, you'll be able to fine-tune your diet, turning your dinner plate into a powerful weapon against disease. Bon appétit.

CHAPTER 1

Fighting Disease With Food

Back in 2697 B.C., a Chinese medical text described a strange disease that left its victims suffering from depression, fatigue, constipation, and numbness or tingling sensations in the legs. Severe cases of the disease, now called *beriberi*, produced heart difficulties, high blood pressure, muscle wasting, and other serious problems. Some forty-five hundred years passed before a very simple cure for beriberi was discovered.

The year A.D. 1735 saw the first known recorded description of another unusual disease, this one striking in Spain, Italy, and later spreading to other parts of the world. This disease, dubbed *pellagra,* caused the "4 Ds": dermatitis, diarrhea, dementia, and eventually death. When pellagra reached epidemic proportions in the southeastern United States, a U.S. government doctor was sent to investigate. He discovered an inexpensive cure that had no side effects.

Beriberi is caused by a lack of thiamin (vitamin B_1). And pellagra results from a deficiency of the B-vitamin called niacin. Both of these serious diseases are prevented or cured by the relatively small amounts of thiamin or niacin found in common foods. And they're not the only ailments associated with the lack of vitamins, minerals, or other substances found in food: Memory difficulties, depression, weak bones, poor wound healing, nerve damage, acne, anemia, gallstones, cracked lips, cataracts, birth defects, numbness of the feet, nausea, anorexia, bleeding gums, easy bruisability, irregular heartbeat, elevated blood pressure, and even cancer have all been linked to a lack of vitamins, minerals, protein, fat, carbohydrates, water, fiber, or any of the hundreds of phytochemicals in foods.

That's the bad news. The good news is that foods supply us with hundreds of known and an untold number of yet-to-be-identified substances that act as medicines, preventing or relieving numerous ailments. One newly appreciated group of these medicinal substances is a "family" of nutrients known as antioxidants/free radical quenchers. The antioxidants and free radical quenchers have generated a lot of excitement in scientific circles, for they appear to be powerful yet natural substances that help the body resist heart disease, stroke, cancer, arthritis, and other debilitating diseases. They do so by controlling oxidation within the body.

Oxidation, or damage caused by oxygen, is a curious phenomenon. Although the oxygen we constantly inhale gives us life, it is also a highly reactive substance that severely damages the body if allowed to "run wild." Imagine what would happen if you left a bicycle outside for a long time. Eventually, the metal would react with oxygen in the air, and the bicycle would rust into uselessness. A similar process occurs within the body. Highly toxic forms of oxygen arise within the body as the byproducts of normal metabolism, or are introduced by exposure to air pollution, cigarette smoke, industrial chemicals, drugs, pesticides, and certain food components. These dangerous particles are called oxidants. Left alone, the oxidants would sweep through the body, "rusting" DNA, cells, and everything else they touch. Little by little over the years, the oxidants attack the nervous system, the circulatory system, the immune system, organs, individual cells, and even the DNA within the cells. It's believed that many diseases, and much of the general deterioration we suffer as we age, are caused by accumulated oxidative damage to the body.

Free radicals, unstable molecules which have lost electrons, are powerful oxidants. Desperately seeking to "balance" themselves, free radicals steal electrons from other molecules. And now that these molecules are missing electrons, they may turn around and snatch electrons from still other molecules. It's like a game of tag, where whoever is touched becomes "it" and must touch someone else. But the free radical touch is dangerously destructive, leading, in the long run, to disease, distress, and aging.

The body protects itself with its own natural antioxidants and free radical quenchers, such as SOD (superoxide dismutase) and glutathione peroxidase. Unfortunately, some people's natural defenses are just not strong enough to control the oxidants and free radicals, especially as the body ages.

Fortunately, the body is assisted by the naturally occurring antioxidants and free radical quenchers in foods. These include beta-carotene, vitamins C and E, the mineral selenium, and more recently identified phytochemicals such as glutathione, lycopene, and quercetin. Many researchers now believe that maintaining high levels of antioxidants and free radical quenchers are the key to preventing heart disease, cancer, arthritis, and other diseases, and to preventing the early onset of aging. And since these substances are found in foods, the healthful diet may be the preferred medicine of the future.

Antioxidants and free radical quenchers are not the only "food medicines." Let's take a look at some common ailments, and the food or nutrients that help to prevent or cure them.

MEDICINAL FOODS HELP FIGHT DISEASE

Acne: A chronic inflammatory skin condition, acne most commonly affects the skin during adolescence, although problems may continue throughout adulthood. Symptoms include "pimples" (small lesions filled with pus), whiteheads, blackheads, cysts, skin redness, and inflammation.

Although chocolate and other foodstuffs have long been blamed for causing acne, none of these claims have stood up to scrutiny. Skin problems in some people may be caused by food allergies, but no single food has been found to cause acne. Instead, oily skin, poor hygiene, certain drugs and cosmetics, a family history of acne, stress, a weakened immune system, and certain endocrine disorders are the more likely pimple-producers.

Foods and Nutrients That Help: Research has shown that yeast may be helpful in combating some cases of acne. Foods containing zinc, such as oysters, wheat germ and lima beans, may also be helpful.

Acquired Immunodeficiency Syndrome (AIDS): Although first identified less than twenty years ago, AIDS quickly became a terrifying condition, striking at the body's ability to resist disease by crippling the immune system. Victims don't die of AIDS itself; instead, they are felled by other diseases that a healthy immune system would normally fend off.

Foods and Nutrients That Help: Although there is no cure for AIDS, early studies suggest that vitamin C may help to slow the spread of the disease. Thus, while not a treatment or cure, the addition of vitamin C-rich foods such as orange juice, strawberries, and Brussels sprouts is a helpful nutritional adjunct in the battle against AIDS.

Some physicians suggest that glutathione peroxidase, an enzyme made by the human body, may also be helpful. Glutathione is a free-radical quencher and antioxidant which helps strengthen the immune system. We can get the nutrients that the body uses to make glutathione, such as selenium, from a variety of common foods, such as seafood, poultry, meat, and whole grains.

Age-related Macular Degeneration (AMD): A common vision problem associated with aging, AMD is caused by progressive deterioration of the macula, which is found right in the center of the retina. It's believed that AMD results from many years' worth of oxidation damage to the macula, but that large amounts of antioxidants will help to prevent the problem.

Foods and Nutrients That Help: The antioxidant vitamins A/beta-carotene, C and E, the minerals selenium and zinc, and other substances such as the anthocyanosides found in blueberries help to prevent AMD. These antioxidants are found in foods such as Alaskan king crab, beet greens, black currants, Brussels sprouts, carrots, cantaloupe, dandelion greens, grapefruit, guava, papaya, mangoes, nuts, oranges, oysters (Eastern), pumpkin, spinach, and wheat germ.

Aging: Although not a disease, aging is often associated with many distressing "symptoms," including loss of memory and strength, poor vision and hearing, lack of energy, and degenerative problems such as arthritis.

Many theories explaining the ravages of aging have been advanced. One of the strongest of these postulates is that the lifelong accumulation of oxidative damage to cells and body tissue is responsible for a great many of the signs and symptoms of aging. In other words, the body is slowly "rusted" by oxidants. This "oxidation theory" argues that eating foods rich in natural antioxidants will help to reduce or slow many of the signs and symptoms of aging by controlling oxidation damage.

Foods and Nutrients That Help: Foods containing good amounts of the antioxidant vitamins A/beta-carotene, C, and E, the mineral selenium, and other natural antioxidant substances should help to hold aging at bay. Such foods include beet greens, black currants, Brussels sprouts, carrots, cantaloupe, dandelion greens, grapefruit, guava, kiwi, papaya, mangoes, nuts, oranges, oysters (Eastern), pumpkin, spinach, and wheat germ.

Garlic may also help the body to resist the effects of aging by detoxifying harmful substances, by protecting cells from the damaging effects of oxidation, by suppressing tumors, and by helping to fight against bacteria and fungi.

Arthritis: Arthritis is a general term referring to inflammation or pain in one or more joints. Severe or constant arthritis pain can limit one's activities and mobility, and has confined many people to wheelchairs or to bed. The most common form of arthritis is osteoarthritis (OA), which is caused by a breakdown of the smooth cartilage that cushions the ends of the bones where they meet to form a joint. As the cartilage deteriorates, the bones rub painfully together. Advanced cases of OA can lead to constant pain that grows worse with time, requiring stronger doses of medicine.

Over 15 million Americans suffer from OA, with almost everyone showing some signs of OA by the age of 65. In addition to pain, typical OA symptoms include stiffness, tenderness, and swelling of the joint(s). Depression is a common side effect of OA.

Foods and Nutrients That Help: The omega-3 fatty acids found in fish have been successfully used to treat patients with

OA, as well as the less common rheumatoid arthritis. Garlic, which helps the body regulate inflammation, also contains sulfur, which has long been known to help with arthritis.

New research suggests that oxidation and free radical damage may cause or worsen some forms of arthritis, so antioxidants and free radical quenchers such as vitamins C and E, beta-carotene, and the mineral selenium may help to prevent or relieve arthritis. Foods high in these nutrients include spinach, carrots, sweet potatoes, hot chili peppers, beet greens, papaya, red peppers, guava, kiwi, asparagus, broccoli, green beans, nuts, whole grains, poultry, and fish.

Atherosclerosis: The hardening of the arteries known as atherosclerosis comes about when cholesterol, fat, platelets, cellular debris, and other substances latch on to the interior walls of the arteries. As the deposits grow in size they become like a dam. They interfere with the flow of blood, and the arteries harden and become less elastic.

If the arteries affected are the coronary arteries, which supply blood to the heart muscle, the result can be angina (chest pain) and a heart attack. If the affected arteries supply blood to the brain, the result may be a stroke.

Atherosclerosis can be combated with foods that help to:

- Lower the total cholesterol and/or the LDL ("bad") cholesterol
- Raise the HDL ("good") cholesterol, which helps to carry cholesterol away from the artery walls
- "Thin" the blood to prevent the formation of unnecessary blood clots that may lodge in partially narrowed arteries

Foods and Nutrients That Help: A variety of foods help to combat atherosclerosis, including alfalfa sprouts, apples, artichokes, asparagus, avocados, barley, beans, blueberries, broccoli, Brussels sprouts, carrots, cantaloupes, cauliflower, celery, fish, garlic, ginger, grapes, mushrooms, nuts, onions, parsley, parsnips, pasta, peas, pears, peppers (hot), prunes, pumpkin, seaweed, spinach, tea, tomatoes, turnips, watermelon, wine, and yeast.

Since the arteries may also be damaged by oxidation and free radicals, antioxidants and free radical quenchers such as vitamins C and E, beta-carotene, and the mineral selenium may help to reduce the risk of atherosclerosis. Foods containing good amounts of antioxidants and free radical quenchers include spinach, carrots, sweet potatoes, hot chili peppers, beet greens, papaya, red peppers, guava, kiwi, asparagus, broccoli, green beans, nuts, whole grains, poultry, and fish.

Cancer: Although actually a group of diseases with varying causes rather than a single disease, for the purposes of discussion cancer can be generally described as the uncontrolled growth of cells within the body. Although the cancer cells themselves may not be deadly, they can interfere with or destroy surrounding cells, tissues, and organs, eventually leading to death.

Foods and Nutrients That Help: Many foods have anticancer properties. Some, like cabbage and broccoli, contain specific anticancer ingredients such as indoles, antioxidants, chlorophyll, and carotenoids. Others, such as rice and barley, are high in fiber, protecting against cancer by limiting the contact between potential carcinogens and the lining of the intestines. Carrots, pumpkins, and other foods rich in vitamins A, C, and E, the mineral selenium, or other natural antioxidants ward off cancer by protecting normal body cells against oxidation damage.

Foods with one or more anticancer properties include apples, apricots, asparagus, avocados, barley, beans, broccoli, Brussels sprouts, cabbage, cantaloupes, carrots, cauliflower, celery, cherries, collard greens, currants, dandelion greens, figs, eggplant, garlic, grapes, grapefruit, guava, kale, kiwi, lemons, lentils, mangoes, mushrooms, nuts, oats, onions, oranges, papaya, parsley, pasta, peppers, potatoes, pumpkin, radishes, rice, rutabaga, seaweed, spinach, strawberries, tangerines, tea, tomatoes, turnips, watercress, watermelon, and wheat.

Cataracts: The clouding of the lens of the eye known as cataracts is a common vision problem afflicting people as they age. Cataracts are caused by hardening of the arteries supplying fresh blood to the vitreous solution surrounding the lens. Nutrients in the blood cannot move through the vitreous solution to the lens, causing it to deteriorate.

In a sense, cataracts are similar to coronary artery disease, which also results when a part of the body is "starved" of nutrients. A good deal of research shows that the damage caused by oxidation and free radicals can also spur the formation of cataracts. Cataracts can be fought by eating foods that:

- Lower the total cholesterol and/or the LDL ("bad") cholesterol
- Raise the HDL ("good") cholesterol, which helps to carry cholesterol away from the artery walls
- Prevent the formation of unnecessary blood clots that may lodge in a partially narrowed artery by "thinning" the blood
- Control the oxidants and free radicals which damage the lenses

Foods and Nutrients That Help: Among the foods that help to keep all the arteries open, including those arteries feeding the eyes, are alfalfa sprouts, apples, artichokes, asparagus, avocados, barley, beans, blueberries, broccoli, Brussels sprouts, cantaloupe, carrots, cauliflower, celery, fish, garlic, ginger, grapes, lentils, lemons, mangoes, mushrooms, nuts, onions, parsley, parsnips, pasta, peas, pears, peppers, prunes, pumpkin, seaweed, spinach, tea, tomatoes, turnips, watermelon, red wine, and yeast. Foods high in antioxidants and free radical quenchers such as vitamins C and E include spinach, carrots, sweet potatoes, hot chili peppers, green peppers, beet greens, papaya, red peppers, guava, kiwi, asparagus, broccoli, green beans, nuts, whole grains, poultry, and fish.

Cholesterol, Elevated: An elevated total cholesterol is a major risk factor for heart disease. Equally troublesome is a high LDL ("bad") cholesterol, or a low HDL ("good") cholesterol. In general, a low-fat, high-fiber diet based on fresh vegetables and fruits, plus whole grains, will help to lower the total cholesterol and LDL, while exercise and moderate amounts of red wine will raise the HDL in many people.

Foods and Nutrients That Help: Foods that help to lower the total cholesterol and LDL, and/or raise the HDL, include alfalfa sprouts, apples, artichokes, avocados, barley, beans, blueberries, carrots, grapefruit, fish, garlic, grapes, grapefruit, guava, kale, lentils, certain nuts, oats (and oat bran), onions, oranges, peas, pears, brown rice (and rice bran), spinach, tangerines, and red wine.

Foods high in soluble fiber are especially helpful. Fiber is a mixture of indigestible substances found in vegetables, grains, and other foods that began their lives as plants. There are two main types of fiber, soluble and insoluble. The soluble fibers found in oat bran, beans, many vegetables, apples, and other foods helps to lower cholesterol. (Insoluble fibers speed the passage of digested foods through the intestines, thus reducing the risk of cancer and promoting regularity.) Although scientists have not yet discovered the exact way in which soluble fiber lowers cholesterol, it appears to interact with bile in the intestines. Instead of being reabsorbed into the body, the "tied up" bile exits the body with the feces. This forces the liver to make more bile—and to use up cholesterol doing so. Many studies have shown that people who eat diets high in soluble fiber, such as oat bran, have lower cholesterol levels than those who do not.

Cold: The common cold is a widespread and contagious infectious viral disease.

Foods and Nutrients That Help: Studies have shown that vitamin C can help to relieve the severity of cold symptoms and the duration of the cold, by stimulating the immune system. Papayas, mangoes, parsley, peppers, and Brussels sprouts are good sources of vitamin C.

Oysters, almonds, and other foods containing zinc may also help in the battle against colds. Zinc inhibits the growth of certain viruses and strengthens the immune system.

It has also been found that eating yogurt may strengthen the immune system and reduce one's susceptibility to colds. One study found that people who ate ¾ cup of yogurt per day suffered from 25 percent fewer colds.

Constipation: Difficult or infrequent bowel movements, and/or producing hard or dry feces are symptoms of constipation. A frequent problem, it may be caused by a low-fiber diet, an inadequate intake of fluids, depression, an anal fissure, tumors, diverticulitis, intestinal obstruction and other problems.

Foods and Nutrients That Help: The simplest and quickest

cure for many cases of constipation is to switch to a high-fiber diet containing foods such as alfalfa sprouts, apples, apricots, barley, beans, beets, broccoli, Brussels sprouts, cabbage, cauliflower, figs, kale, lentils, mangoes, papayas, peaches, prunes, popcorn, raspberries, rhubarb, whole-grain rice, and whole-grain wheat.

Drinking 8 glasses of water a day as you increase your fiber intake is extremely important for water lubricates the digestive tract and the mucus membranes lining it.

Diabetes: Non-insulin–dependent diabetes (also known as NIDDM or adult-onset diabetes) is a metabolic problem often seen in overweight adults. Either their bodies are not producing enough insulin to control their blood sugars, or insulin receptors on their cells have been altered and do not respond to the insulin's attempt to push sugar into the cells.

Diabetes can cause frequent urination, excessive thirst and hunger, fatigue, decreased resistance to disease, as well as damage to the nerves, kidneys, and circulatory system. Blood vessels harmed by diabetes may function poorly, causing a "second round" of damage to many parts of the body, including the heart and the eyes. Damage to the nerves may result in numbness, burning and tingling sensations in the feet and hands, or in gangrene and amputation of a limb. Kidney failure is another danger of diabetes.

Foods and Nutrients That Help: Onions, garlic, beans, lentils, fish, barley, broccoli, plus other foods high in protein and fiber can assist in preventing or ameliorating adult-onset diabetes by helping to control blood sugar.

Diarrhea: The loose, watery bowel movements of diarrhea, sometimes accompanied by abdominal pain and lack of bowel control, may be caused by infections, stress, emotional upset, lactose intolerance ("milk allergy"), certain drugs, too many prunes or other foods, malabsorption syndrome, irritable bowel syndrome, tumors in the gastrointestinal tract, and other problems.

Foods and Nutrients That Help: If the diarrhea is caused by lactose intolerance, avoiding all milk and milk products should solve the problem. Otherwise, low-fiber foods such as cottage cheese, saltine-type crackers, mashed potatoes, and well-cooked rice with rice water are helpful. Eating these and other low-fiber foods gives the intestines little bulk to "push" against, slowing the peristalsis (contractions) that normally move the food ahead. Chicken broth offers a great deal of nourishment with no fiber. Pectin-rich foods such as pears and apples can help to solidify the stools (especially if you remove the skins before eating, to reduce the fiber load). In addition, blueberry soup (made from dried blueberries) has long been recommended by doctors in Sweden. Most likely, blueberry soup works because it contains proanthocyanidins, which help to kill the bacteria *E. coli* which may be causing the diarrhea. Yogurt is also helpful, as are bananas, which promote the growth of helpful bacteria in the bowel.

Digestion, Poor: Many people are plagued by heartburn, excess gas, rumbling in the stomach and other digestive upsets. Figs, garlic and papaya have all been successfully used as aids to minor digestive problems. Garlic is especially helpful in destroying intestinal parasites.

Diverticular Disease: Small, sac-like swellings that arise in the wall of the colon are called diverticula, and the inflammation of these is called diverticulitis. Symptoms of diverticular disease include abdominal tenderness or cramping, constipation, fever, and nausea.

Foods and Nutrients That Help: Although there is no guaranteed method of preventing diverticular disease, eating a high-fiber diet and avoiding straining when eliminating reduce the risk. Foods that are high in fiber and/or reduce straining include alfalfa sprouts, apples, apricots, barley, beans, beets, broccoli, Brussels sprouts, cabbage, cauliflower, papayas, popcorn, raspberries, rhubarb, whole-grain rice and whole-grain wheat.

Headaches: The pain associated with a "tension" or "stress" headache is annoying, but not usually debilitating. Less common is the intense pain of a migraine headache, which may be accompanied by nausea and vomiting,

Foods and Nutrients That Help: The omega-3 fatty acids found in fish such as salmon, mackerel, and sardines may reduce the frequency and/or severity of migraine headaches.

Heart Disease: Although we normally think of "heart attacks" when heart disease is mentioned, there are other heart problems, including irregular heartbeat and congestive heart failure.

Irregular Heart Rhythms: Electrical current generated in the heart keeps the heart muscle beating rhythmically. Potentially fatal problems can arise if the rhythm becomes too fast (tachycardia), slow (bradycardia), or irregular (arrhythmia).

Foods and Nutrients That Help: Potassium-rich foods such as bananas, peanuts, and potatoes help to keep the heart beating rhythmically.

Coronary Heart Disease: The leading cause of death in the United States, coronary heart disease is really just a "plumbing" problem. There are no germs involved. Instead, the arteries supplying the heart muscle with fresh blood become blocked. Blood flow dries up, and part or all of the heart muscle dies of "starvation." The result is a heart attack, which may be fatal.

Coronary artery disease can be fought by eating plenty of foods that:

• Lower the total cholesterol and/or the LDL ("bad") cholesterol
• Raise the HDL ("good") cholesterol which helps to carry cholesterol away from the artery walls
• Prevent the formation of unnecessary blood clots that may lodge in a partially narrowed artery by "thinning" the blood
• Control free radical damage, which can encourage the formation of plaque by damaging artery walls

Foods and Nutrients That Help: There are many heart-healthy foods which help to keep cholesterol, oxidation, and free radical damage under control. These include alfalfa sprouts, apples, artichokes, asparagus, avocados, barley, beans, blueberries, broccoli, Brussels sprouts, cantaloupes, carrots, cauliflower, celery, fish, garlic, ginger, grapes, lentils, lemons, mangoes, mushrooms, nuts, onions, parsley, parsnips, pasta, peas, pears, peppers, prunes, pumpkin, seaweed, spinach, tea, tomatoes, turnips, watermelon, red wine, and yeast.

Beta-carotene, vitamins C and E, and the mineral selenium

can help to prevent the oxidation and free radical damage that can encourage heart disease. Spinach, carrots, sweet potatoes, hot chili peppers, beet greens, papaya, red peppers, guava, kiwi, asparagus, broccoli, green beans, nuts, whole grains, poultry, and fish contain good amounts of these antioxidant and free radical quenching nutrients.

Herpes Simplex: Caused by a contagious virus, herpes simplex causes "cold sores" on the lips, gums, genitals, and, in rare cases, the cornea of the eye. Herpes thrives in the presence of an amino acid called arginine. Foods containing another amino acid, lysine, "balance out" arginine, canceling the "helping hand" arginine gives to the disease.

Foods and Nutrients That Help: Eating fewer foods that contain arginine, such as nuts and seeds, while eating more foods containing lysine, such as buckwheat, milk, and soybeans, may help to control herpes. Other foods, such as seaweed and strawberries, also contain substances with anti-herpes properties.

Hemorrhoids: Also known as "piles," hemorrhoids are dilated veins in the rectum or anus. They can cause pain, itching, and bleeding. Larger hemorrhoids can leave you feeling as if you still "have to go" after moving your bowels. Hemorrhoids may be caused by constipation, straining to eliminate, obesity, pregnancy, anal intercourse, and rectal surgery.

Foods and Nutrients That Help: Hemorrhoids caused by constipation and straining to eliminate can be prevented by eating foods that ease the process of elimination. Such foods include alfalfa sprouts, apples, apricots, barley, beans, beets, broccoli, Brussels sprouts, bran, cabbage, cauliflower, papayas, popcorn, raspberries, rhubarb, rice, whole-grain rice, and whole-grain wheat.

Hypertension: Hypertension (high blood pressure) seems to strike "naturally" as we age, but studies of large population groups have shown that there is nothing natural about it. A primary risk factor for heart disease, high blood pressure can often be prevented or controlled through nutritional means, coupled with lifestyle changes, exercise, stress reduction and, sometimes, medication.

Foods and Nutrients That Help: The standard American high-fat, low-fiber diet is linked to elevated blood pressure. Foods that are low in fat and high in fiber may help to combat the problem. A diet based on a variety of fresh vegetables and whole-grains (avoiding fatty avocados and olives) fits the bill.

Diets high in sodium (salt) have also been linked to hypertension. Since the mineral potassium "cancels out" some of sodium's effects, eating foods high in potassium may help to prevent high blood pressure. Bananas, peanuts, and blueberries are among the foods with the largest amounts of potassium.

The omega-3 fats found in fish such as mackerel, sardines, and salmon may also help to lower blood pressure, as do garlic and okra. In addition, celery contains 3-n-butylphthalide, while garlic and onions contain organic sulfur compounds such as allicin and diallyl disulfide, which apparently lower blood pressure.

Immune Deficiency: The body's own "department of defense," the immune system, fights off cancer, bacteria, viruses, and other dangerous substances that invade or arise within the body. Immune-system weakness can lead to a host of problems, ranging from mild colds to deadly cancer.

Foods and Nutrients That Help: Like any other army, the immune system travels on its stomach, and needs as many nutrient-rich foods as possible in order to stay in good shape. Although all of the nutrients, from vitamin A to zinc, help to keep the immune system strong, some are especially helpful. Vitamin A, also called the "anti-infection vitamin," strengthens the immune system in the respiratory and digestive tracts, the skin, eyes and other parts of the body that are the first to be "hit" by invading germs. Vitamin B_6 keeps the thymus gland, where the germ-fighting T-cells are "schooled," strong. The body must have plentiful supplies of vitamin B_{12} and folic acid in order for immune-system cells to grow to powerful maturity in the bone marrow. Vitamin C energizes the disease-fighting T-cells and B-cells, while strengthening the large macrophages ("cell eaters"), which literally swallow and destroy bacteria, viruses, and other substances that cause disease. Of the many minerals, zinc has perhaps the most powerful effect upon the immune system. It helps to ensure that the thymus gland remains healthy, that there are enough T-cells to engage invaders in hand-to-hand combat, and that the B-cells can produce antibodies. An enzyme named glutathione peroxidase, which is a powerful antioxidant and free radical quencher, assists the immune system in keeping us healthy. The body manufactures its own glutathione, but needs nutrients such as selenium from foods in order to do so.

All foods contain nutrients that aid the immune system. Strong immune-boosting foods include: broccoli, cabbage, garlic, grapes, grapefruit, guava, kale, lemons, mushrooms, oysters, papayas, pineapple, pumpkin, seaweed, tangerines, and yogurt.

Infection: Infections arise when viruses, bacteria, or parasites invade the body, possibly damaging body tissue and triggering a massive response from the immune system. The resulting battle between the immune system and the invaders may cause inflammation and damage to body tissue.

Foods and Nutrients That Help: Apples, bananas, barley, blueberries, cabbage, celery, cranberries, garlic, ginger, grapes, licorice, mushrooms, onions, oranges, papaya, raspberries, seaweed, tea, and yogurt are among the foods with anti-infection properties. Blueberries and cranberries are especially effective against bladder infections.

Infertility, Male: In order for a man to be potent, he must have adequate amounts of healthy, "frisky" sperm that can survive the difficult trip through a woman's reproductive system and fertilize an egg.

Foods and Nutrients That Help: Vitamin C and the mineral zinc have both been shown to help keep a man's sperm strong and healthy. Foods high in vitamin C or zinc include chicken liver, oranges, oysters, papayas, red peppers, spinach, strawberries, tomatoes, and wheat germ.

Insomnia: Difficulty falling or staying asleep, and/or early-morning wakefulness are symptoms of insomnia, the most common sleep disorder. Depression, anxiety, pain, erratic work hours, certain medications, an over-active thyroid gland, emotional stress, disturbances in brain function, or drug dependence and abuse can cause insomnia.

Foods and Nutrients That Help: Vitamin B_6 and niacin are necessary for normal sleep. If the insomnia is due to a deficiency of either of these two vitamins, then adding foods such as bananas, barley, buckwheat, cantaloupe, beans, almonds, whole-grain rice, and whole-grain wheat may remedy the deficiency and solve the problem.

If the insomnia is not related to a lack of the two vitamins, then foods containing tryptophan may be helpful. Tryptophan is a naturally occurring amino acid which the body converts to a sleep-inducing neurotransmitter called serotonin. Tryptophan-rich foods that may help those suffering from short-term insomnia include bananas, cheese, milk, pasta, and turkey.

Mental Slowness: Deficiencies in a number of nutrients, including amino acids, such as l-phenylalanine, may contribute to poor mental functioning.

Foods and Nutrients That Help: A lack of vitamin B_1 has been associated with a slowing of brain activity. Brewer's yeast, wheat germ, peas, and carrots are good sources of B_1.

Good amounts of vitamin B_2 (5–10 milligrams per day) seem to encourage a better memory. Mushrooms, spinach, brewer's yeast, and beet greens contain good amounts of B_2.

Beta-carotene has been associated with strong cognitive (thinking) skills. Good sources of beta-carotene include carrots, parsley, apricots, spinach, and pumpkin.

A little-known mineral named boron plays an important role in mental alertness. Boron apparently helps to stimulate and/ or regulate electrical activity in the brain. Studies have shown that a low-boron diet leads to a slowdown in electrical activity and a decrease in mental performance. The problem is cured when good amounts of the mineral are restored to the diet. Apples, broccoli, grapes, nuts and peaches all contain boron.

Menopause: Menopause signals the end of menstruation in women. Menopausal women may suffer from hot flashes, vaginal dryness, weight gain, irregular periods, varicose veins, sleep disturbances, enlargement or shrinkage of the breasts, and other symptoms to varying degrees.

Foods and Nutrients That Help: Boron can help to boost a woman's estrogen levels and reduce or relieve many of the symptoms of menopause. Foods containing boron or other substances with estrogenic properties include apples, broccoli,

Brussels sprouts, cabbage, carrots, dates, grapes, legumes, nuts, oats, peanuts, raisins, and soy products.

Motion Sickness: Ginger helps to relieve the temporary stomach upset, dizziness, and general feeling of malaise that strikes some people when they are driving, flying, or boating.

Obesity: Scientists do not know exactly why people accumulate excess body fat. Some cases may have a biochemical basis, while others may be due to unhealthy lifestyles.

Foods and Nutrients That Help: Although there is no cure for obesity, apples and whole wheat help to curb the appetite by giving one a full feeling. Some studies suggest that eating mustard, ginger, hot peppers, and other hot and spicy foods can "rev up" the metabolism and burn off calories.

Osteoporosis: The "thinning of the bones" that often afflicts many women after menopause is called osteoporosis. It's estimated that some 15 million Americans have osteoporosis, the most common of all bone diseases. The bones of the legs, spine, pelvis, and jaw, as well as the teeth, slowly become thin and brittle, and may break easily. Unfortunately, the problem is often symptomless until the advanced stages of the disease, and a woman may not know that she has osteoporosis until she slips and breaks her hip. By then, it's much too late to do anything about it.

Foods and Nutrients That Help: A lifelong diet of foods rich in calcium, vitamin D, boron, and other vitamins and minerals can help to keep the bones as strong as possible for as long as possible. Milk and other nonfat dairy products, canned salmon with the bones, soy products, apples, prunes and nuts are among the foods that help to keep bones strong.

Regular weight-bearing exercises such as walking, running, and lifting weights also help to keep bones strong by "stressing" them. This "stress" signals the body to stop pulling minerals out of the bones. Studies have shown that regular weight-bearing exercise can even increase bone mass. Estrogen replacement therapy (ERT) is also used to help keep bones strong in menopausal women.

Respiratory Ailments: Colds, asthma, bronchitis, and other common respiratory ailments make breathing difficult for millions and they can be quite severe. Asthma, for example, can require medication and hospitalization. If not controlled, it can lead to emphysema, permanent obstructive lung disease, and death.

Foods and Nutrients That Help: "Hot" foods such as garlic, onions, mustard, and chili may help to make breathing easier. Garlic acts as a decongestant to open up blocked airways, an expectorant to help one cough up mucus, and an antispasmodic to calm the bronchial spasms associated with asthma and other respiratory problems. (Bronchial spasms interfere with the flow of air through the air passages, just as a hand squeezing tightly on a hose can make it difficult for water to get through.)

Onions help to reduce bronchial inflammation, and have antihistamine properties. Mustard and chili can help to clear away the mucus which clogs up the airways.

Skin Diseases: Both eczema and psoriasis are common, chronic skin disorders. With eczema, the skin becomes thickened and develops scales. Small blisters appear and may ooze, and the skin is itchy. Psoriasis can produce itching in the affected area, joint pain, and raised patches of skin covered with large silver-white or white scales.

Foods and Nutrients That Help: Omega-3 fish oils, whether eaten in foods or taken as supplements, have shown promise in fighting eczema, psoriasis, and other skin problems, as well as reducing inflammation, itching, scaling, and skin sensitivity. Mackerel, herring, sablefish, salmon, whitefish, and other fish contain the omega-3s.

Stroke: Also known as a cerebrovascular accident, a stroke is much like a heart attack in that there is a sudden interruption to the blood flow. But in this case, it's brain tissue that suffers, not heart muscle. Strokes can be caused by a narrowing or complete blockage in an artery supplying blood to the brain, or by a blood clot lodging in an artery. A break in a brain artery, allowing blood to seep into the surrounding brain tissue, can also cause a stroke.

Foods and Nutrients That Help: The same foods that prevent coronary heart disease can also protect against strokes by keeping the arteries to the brain open and the blood flowing—foods that help to:

• Prevent unnecessary blood clots by "thinning" the blood
• Lower the total cholesterol and/or the LDL ("bad") cholesterol
• Raise the HDL ("good") cholesterol, which helps to carry cholesterol away from the artery walls
• Control the free radical damage which can encourage the formation of plaque by damaging artery walls

These foods include alfalfa sprouts, apples, artichokes, asparagus, avocados, bananas, barley, beans, blueberries, broccoli, Brussels sprouts, carrots, cantaloupe, cauliflower, celery, fish, garlic, ginger, grapes, kale, mushrooms, nuts, onions, parsley, parsnips, pasta, peas, pears, hot peppers, prunes, pumpkin, seaweed, spinach, tea, tomatoes, turnips, watermelon, red wine, and yeast.

Foods that contain vitamins C and E, beta-carotene, selenium, and other substances which control oxidation and free radical damage also help to prevent strokes by keeping the arteries to the brain strong and clear. Spinach, carrots, sweet potatoes, hot chili peppers, beet greens, papaya, red peppers, guava, kiwi, asparagus, broccoli, green beans, nuts, whole grains, poultry, and fish contain good amounts of these and other substances that control oxidation and free radical damage.

Ulcers: These small erosions in the lining of the gastrointestinal tract may produce pain, loss of appetite and weight, bloody stool, and vomiting. The exact symptoms depend upon what part of the gastrointestinal tract is involved.

Although bland, low-fiber diets and milk were once thought to be necessary for ulcer patients, new research has discovered that the old diet is actually harmful. A high-fiber diet is better.

Foods and Nutrients That Help: Bananas, cabbage, figs, licorice, seaweed, tea, and wheat may all prevent or soothe ulcers. Some evidence even suggests that eating hot peppers may protect the stomach against ulcers. If you already have ulcers, however, do not eat hot peppers or anything else that causes pain or distress.

Varicose Veins: The bluish, enlarged veins snaking their way under skin are called varicose veins. They can appear in many parts of the body, even the esophagus, but are usually found in the legs or anus (where they are called hemorrhoids). Pregnancy, previous vein disease, and standing for long periods of time are some of the common causes of varicose veins. Prolonged straining when moving the bowels also contributes to varicose veins in the legs, and to hemorrhoids.

    Foods and Nutrients That Help: Eating foods which soften the stool and eliminate straining may help prevent varicose veins. Such foods include alfalfa sprouts, apples, apricots, barley, beans, beets, broccoli, Brussels sprouts, cabbage, cauliflower, papaya, popcorn, raspberries, rhubarb, whole-grain rice, and whole-grain wheat.

CHAPTER 2

What Vitamins Do for You

Vitamins are a group of compounds that we need in small amounts to remain healthy. Otherwise, the thirteen recognized vitamins are not all related to one another, are not all from the same chemical "family," and do not all have similar functions or structures. The primary link between the various vitamins is that they are absolutely essential for growth, health and life, and that we cannot make them, or enough of them, ourselves, inside our bodies. Instead, we must get vitamins from our foods.

The vitamins are divided into two categories: Water-soluble and fat-soluble. The water-soluble vitamins (vitamins B_1, B_2, B_6, B_{12}, biotin, folic acid, niacin, pantothenic acid, and C) are found in the watery portions of food. Since they are only stored in the body in small amounts, we should eat foods containing these vitamins daily. Their fat-soluble counterparts (vitamins A, D, E, and K) are absorbed from food along with the fats in the food, and are stored in the body. Although they are found in foods, vitamins themselves do not supply calories that we can burn for energy, or fat to store for future use, or protein to build body tissues.

Although the first vitamin, A, was not discovered until 1913, for centuries we'd been aware of what happens when vitamins are lacking in a diet. Perhaps the most famous case of vitamin deficiency involved scurvy, the scourge of explorers, travelers, and warriors who ate no fresh fruits or vegetables for long periods of time. The Crusaders marching from Europe to Jerusalem in the eleventh, twelfth, and thirteenth centuries were often defeated not by the enemy, but by the symptoms of scurvy: weakness, shortness of breath, bones that fractured easily, wounds that failed to heal, pain, hysteria, depression, swelling and inflammation of the gums, and other ailments. The same problems later afflicted British sailors aboard ship for long ocean voyages. Often, one-half or more of the poor sailors would die of scurvy.

Scurvy was not cured until the late 1700s, when the Dutch Navy began feeding its sailors citrus fruit, and the British Navy gave their sailing men limes and lemons to eat. An unknown factor in the citrus fruit, which we now know is vitamin C, prevented scurvy. It was that simple. A microscopic amount of a vitamin inside a lime was all it took to conquer the killer scurvy, and to give British sailors a nickname that has endured since: "Limeys."

Since the discovery of vitamin A, twelve more vitamins have been identified, and their tasks explained. Let's take a quick look at the vitamins, their uses, properties, and sources. You'll find a chart of the RDAs (Recommended Daily Allowances) for these vitamins at the end of this chapter.

THE VITAMINS

Vitamin A/Beta-Carotene

Also called the "anti-inflammation vitamin" and the "skin vitamin," vitamin A was the first of the vitamins to be discovered, back in 1913.

Vitamin A is really a group of related substances with vitamin A–like activity. Retinol, retinal, beta-carotene, and other carotenoids are all members of the "vitamin A family." Vitamin A, or "preformed vitamin A," is the "animal form" of the vitamin found in liver and other foods that come from animals. Beta-carotene, or "provitamin A," is the "plant form" of the vitamin. Found in vegetables and other foods that come from plants, beta-carotene, one of some 400 members of the carotene family, is converted to vitamin A as needed inside the body.

Vitamin A's Duties: Vitamin A/beta-carotene helps to keep

the immune system strong; promotes fertility; is necessary for protein synthesis; and helps to keep the skin, respiratory tract, esophagus, stomach, intestine, colon, rectum, kidney, urinary tract, and gall bladder healthy.

Various studies suggest that vitamin A and/or beta-carotene may prevent cancers of the stomach, colon, rectum, bladder, breast, mouth, esophagus, cervix, and lungs; act as an antioxidant to guard against heart disease and stroke; and prevent premature aging of the skin. Vitamin A is essential for healthy eyes, as well as successful pregnancy and lactation. It helps the body resist infection, and is required for the formation of bones and growth.

Harvard researchers who studied 90,000 nurses for eight years found that eating beta-carotene–rich foods can reduce the risk of having a stroke by as much as 40 percent. A study conducted in Belgium, which focused on people who had just suffered strokes, found that the odds of survival were better among those who had higher levels of vitamin A/beta-carotene in their blood. This may be because vitamin A/beta-carotene reduces the oxidation damage to nerve cells that occurs as a result of a stroke. With more nerve and other cells intact, the odds of recovering are improved.

The "Physicians's Healthy Study" and the "Beta-Carotene and Retinol Efficacy Trial," two major studies which published their results in 1995, have raised questions concerning the value of taking vitamin A or beta-carotene supplements for cancer. Although the results of these studies are intriguing, they are concerned with supplements, not the nutrients we get from food. No one doubts the tremendous value of the beta-carotene and vitamin A we get from our food.

Deficiency Signs and Symptoms: A deficiency may cause susceptibility to recurrent infections, night blindness, skin and other problems. Three major nutrition studies conducted in the 1970s and 1980s found that 20 percent or more of Americans were taking in less than 70 percent of the RDA for vitamin A.

Where To Find It and Other Vital Information: Vitamin A is found in foods of animal origin, such as butter, milk, and liver. Beta-carotene, the plant form of the vitamin, is found in yellow and orange vegetables and fruits, as well as in dark green, leafy vegetables. Any disorder that interferes with the absorption of fat in the intestines, such as Crohn's Disease, can disrupt the absorption of vitamin A/beta-carotene from food.

Selected Sources of Beta-Carotene

Food	Serving Size	Beta-Carotene (IU)
Sweet potatoes	4 oz, baked	2,488
Carrots	1 raw	2,025
Spinach	½ c, boiled	737
Butternut squash	½ c cubes, baked	714
Dandelion greens	½ c, chopped, cooked	608
Watercress	10 sprigs	490
Chili peppers, hot	1 raw	484
Kale	½ c, chopped, cooked	481
Turnip greens	½ c, chopped, boiled	396
Beet greens	½ c, boiled	367

Biotin

Biotin was actually the first vitamin to be discovered, in 1901. This was in the early days of vitamin research, however, before we really understood vitamins, so this strange new substance was given the name "bios," meaning "life." Biotin was "discovered" again through the years by other researchers who thought they were finding something new. It was named "protective factor X," "coenzyme R," and "vitamin H" before researchers realized that all of these substances were the same thing, which they renamed biotin. We get this member of the B-family of vitamins from a variety of foods. It is also manufactured by intestinal bacteria.

Biotin's Duties: Biotin plays a role in many body systems. It is vital for a strong immune system; necessary for healthy skin, hair, nerves, sex glands, and bone marrow; and is used by the body to turn protein, fat, and carbohydrates into energy.

Deficiency Signs and Symptoms: A deficiency of biotin, which is rare, may lead to skin problems, nausea and vomiting, exhaustion, hair loss, depression, chest and muscle pains, an increase in cholesterol level, and liver enlargement.

Where to Find It and Other Vital Information: Bacteria in our intestines manufacture biotin. We also get the vitamin from egg yolk, nuts, brewer's yeast, soybeans, oatmeal, bananas, mushrooms, and cauliflower.

Long-term use of antibiotics, oral contraceptives or estrogen replacement therapy may cause a biotin deficiency. We should eat foods containing this vitamin daily, for little is stored in the body.

Selected Sources of Biotin

Food	Serving Size	Biotin (mcg)
Beef liver	3½ oz, cooked	96
Soybeans	3½ oz, cooked	61
Rice bran	3½ oz	60
Peanut butter	3½ oz	39
Barley	3½ oz, cooked	31
Oatmeal	3½ oz, cooked	24

Folic Acid
(Also known as folacin and folate)

This member of the B-family of vitamins might have been named "spinachium" because it was originally extracted from the spinach leaf in 1941. Instead, it was named after the Latin word for leaf, *folium.*

Folic acid is actually a family of related compounds, rather than a single substance. We get most of our folic acid from our foods, but some is manufactured by intestinal bacteria.

Folic Acid's Duties: Folic acid regulates cell division and helps maintain DNA and RNA; it is also essential for a strong immune system. Folic acid may prevent cancer of the cervix by curtailing the transformation of normal cells into cancerous ones and by helping them repair themselves.

Deficiency Signs and Symptoms: Lack of folic acid can lead to anemia, problems with digestion, malnutrition, weakness, forgetfulness, diarrhea, vomiting, poor growth in children, and birth defects.

Folic acid deficiencies have also been linked to an easy fatigability, which clears up when the deficiency is corrected. In one study, four people complaining of easy fatigability and other symptoms were found to have low levels of folic acid. When they were given folic acid supplements, their levels of the vitamin rose and their fatigue disappeared. Another study looked at 38 patients suffering from fatigue, depression, burning feet, and other problems. When given 10 milligrams of folic acid per day for 2 to 3 months, their symptoms cleared up.

Pregnant women, or women who intend to become pregnant, should make sure that they are getting enough folic acid, which the fetus needs in order to properly form and close up the neural tube. Otherwise, the child may be born with spina bifida or other serious defects. Because the neural tube closes very early in pregnancy, often before a woman knows that she is carrying a child, the U.S. Public Health Service suggests that women planing to become pregnant should make sure that they are getting at least 0.4 milligrams of folic acid daily. The elderly, who are often deficient in folic acid, should also make sure that their diets contain plenty of dark green leafy vegetables and other foods rich in folic acid.

Where to Find It and Other Vital Information: Folic acid is found in many foods, including dark green, leafy vegetables, brewer's yeast, liver, beets, avocado, broccoli, and orange juice. Folic acid's enemies are stress, alcoholism, and disease. Aspirin, oral contraceptives and numerous other medicines can hamper the body's ability to use the vitamin. Heat, food processing, and excessive boiling can reduce the folic acid content of foods. We should eat foods containing this vitamin daily, for little is stored in the body.

Selected Sources of Folic Acid

Food	Serving Size	Folic Acid (mcg)
Liver	3 oz, cooked	185
Lentils	½ c, boiled	179
Pinto beans	½ c, boiled	146
Adzuki beans	½ c, boiled	139
Black beans	½ c, boiled	128
Asparagus, canned	½ c, spears	116
Kidney beans	½ c, boiled	114
Spinach	½ c, cooked	131
Chicory	½ c, chopped raw	99
Turnip greens	½ c, boiled chopped	85
Lettuce, Romaine	1 c, shredded	76
Avocado	3 oz	62
Papaya	5 ½ oz	58
Parsley	½ c, chopped raw	55

Niacin

The discovery of niacin sprang from an effort to cure a widespread, devastating illness that afflicted the southern parts of the United States. The disease, called pellagra, caused its victims to suffer from a variety of problems, including confusion, memory loss, weakness, diarrhea, and blotchy skin rashes.

A U.S. Bureau of Public Health doctor realized that the problem had to do with poor diet, specifically a diet high in processed cornmeal, which was low in niacin. The devastating epidemic of pellagra was cured when foods containing niacin or the amino acid tryptophan (which the body can convert to niacin) were added to the diet.

Niacin's Duties: Niacin, a member of the B-family of vitamins, is vital for the health and maintenance of the skin, mouth, intestines, and nerves. The body uses niacin to extract energy from carbohydrates, protein, and fat.

Scientists studying cancer feel that niacin helps normal cells resist the changes that turn them cancerous. Niacin can also help the heart. In high doses, niacin supplements (in the form of nicotinic acid) lower the total cholesterol, the LDL (''bad'') cholesterol and the blood fats, while raising the HDL ("good") cholesterol.

Deficiency Signs and Symptoms: A lack of niacin can cause problems such as headaches, muscle weakness, fatigue, nausea and vomiting, irritability, skin dryness, and scales. A severe deficiency produces the "4Ds" of pellagra: dermatitis, diarrhea, dementia, and eventually death. The elderly are at risk of deficiency, even if their diets contain adequate amounts of the vitamin, because the ability to absorb nutrients from food often drops as we age.

Where to Find It and Other Vital Information: Good sources of niacin include chicken, fish, peanut butter, milk and cheese, nuts, liver, and fortified grains and cereals. Since the amino acid tryptophan can be converted by the body into niacin, milk and other foods high in tryptophan are also considered good sources of niacin. Niacin in foods is not significantly affected by exposure to light, heat, or air. Small amounts of niacin leach out into cooking water and are lost if the cooking water is discarded. We should eat foods containing this vitamin daily, for little is stored in the body.

Selected Sources of Niacin

Food	Serving Size	Niacin (mg)
Chicken breast	3 oz, meat only	11.8
Turkey, white meat	3 oz, meat only, roasted	5.8
Beef liver	3 oz, braised	9.1
Salmon, canned	3 oz	6.5
Mackerel, canned	3 oz	8.9
Barley, pearled	1 c, dry	7.4
Bulgur	1 c, dry parboiled	7.4
Peaches, dried	10 halves	5.7
Avocado, Florida	1	5.9

Pantothenic Acid

Named after *pantos,* the Greek word for "everywhere," pantothenic acid is widely available in foods of both plant and animal origin.

Pantothenic Acid's Duties: As part of coenzyme A, pantothenic acid helps to break down carbohydrates, protein, and fats to use for energy. It also plays a role in the manufacture of red blood cells, hormones, neurotransmitters, cholesterol, and vitamin D.

Studies have shown that pantothenic acid supplements can lower cholesterol by up to 15 percent, and reduce triglycerides (blood fats) by as much as 20 to 30 percent in people with high blood fat levels. Some proponents have also argued that taking pantothenic acid can improve athletic ability.

Deficiency Signs and Symptoms: Deficiencies of pantothenic acid are unknown because the vitamin is so readily available in foods. A deficiency can be created under laboratory conditions by feeding volunteers special diets low in pantothenic acid, and by giving them a drug that "cancels out" the vitamin. Suffering from an artificial deficiency, the volunteers complained of skin problems, pains in the arms and legs, fainting, nausea, loss of appetite, depression, lack of coordination, upper respiratory infections, poor healing of wounds, and rapid pulse.

Where to Find It and Other Vital Information: Pantothenic acid is found in whole-grain cereals, nuts, peas, green leafy vegetables, brewer's yeast, and other common foods. The pantothenic acid content of food may be severely depleted by cooking, freezing, and thawing. Processing and canning of other foods also lowers the amounts of this vitamin. We must eat foods containing this vitamin regularly, for little is stored in the body.

Selected Sources of Pantothenic Acid

Food	Serving Size	Pantothenic Acid (mg)
Calf's liver	3½ oz, cooked	11.0
Peanuts	3½ oz	2.8
Mushrooms	3½ oz	2.2
Lentils	3½ oz, cooked	1.4
Broccoli	3½ oz	1.2
Brown rice	3½ oz, cooked	1.1
Cauliflower	3½ oz, cooked	1.0

Vitamin B₁
(Also known as thiamin)

What researchers originally dubbed "vitamin B," turned out to be a series of vitamins, which were christened "B₁," "B₂," "B₃," and so on as they were separated from the original "vitamin B."

Vitamin B₁'s Duties: Vitamin B₁ is necessary for healthy functioning of every cell in the body, especially nerve cells. B₁ assists in the breakdown and conversion of fats, protein, and carbohydrates to energy. Recent studies have suggested that B₁ plays a role in the prevention of cataracts.

Deficiency Signs and Symptoms: Symptoms of deficiency include numbness and weakness in the arms and legs, constipation, burning sensations in the feet, heart enlargement, slowing of the heartbeat, memory loss, confusion, and depression. The classic B₁ deficiency disease is beriberi, a disease that primarily strikes groups whose diets are based on polished rice (from which the B₁ has been removed).

Since B₁ plays an important role in the metabolism of many substances within body cells, a lack of B₁ may lead to the accumulation of "debris" within the cells. If so, the B₁ deficiency symptoms may be caused by the cells becoming overloaded with "trash."

Where to Find It and Other Vital Information: Vitamin B₁ is found in peanuts, pork, fresh and dried peas, oranges, dried beans, whole-grain breads, fortified breads, and rice. A diet high in sugar and refined foods may deplete one's supply of B₁. Excessive cooking of food, or exposing the food to heat or air, can reduce the amount of B₁. Vitamin B₁ deficiency is common among alcoholics. We must eat foods containing this vitamin regularly, for little is stored in the body.

Selected Sources of Vitamin B₁

Food	Serving Size	Vitamin B₁ (mg)
Sunflower seeds, dried	1 oz	.7
Orange juice	6 oz, frozen, reconstituted	.6
Bulgur parboiled	1 c, dried	.5
Spinach noodles	1 c, cooked	.4
Pine nuts, dried	1 oz	.4
Hickory nuts, dried	1 oz	.3
Yellow corn	1 ear, boiled	.2
Potato	7 oz, baked	.2

Vitamin B₂
(Also known as riboflavin)

B₂ is a yellow, fluorescent substance that gives urine its characteristic color. B₂ is easily absorbed in the intestines. The process works better when food is present, so B₂ is better absorbed from foods than it is from supplements. (If you take B₂ supplements, you should take them with meals for the same reason.)

Vitamin B₂'s Duties: Like B₁, vitamin B₂ plays an important role in the body's breakdown and usage of fats, protein, and carbohydrates. B₂ also helps to produce red blood cells and certain hormones, and is necessary for the manufacture and repair of body tissues.

Deficiency Signs and Symptoms: Early signs of B₂ deficiency include burning and itching of the eyes, problems with vision, burning and soreness of the tongue, mouth and lips, and cracks around the corners of the mouth. Symptoms of a more severe B₂ deficiency include depression, hysteria, inflammation of the mucous membranes of the mouth, greasy scaling of the skin, and other skin problems. Pregnant women deficient in B₂ may give birth to malformed children, or children whose growth is retarded.

Where to Find It and Other Vital Information: Liver, milk and milk products are excellent sources of B₂. Yogurt, beef, fortified cereals and breads, broccoli, spinach and other green vegetables also contain the vitamin. Cooking does not harm

B_2, and relatively little is lost to the cooking water when boiling or steaming. Light, however, destroys the B_2 in food, and excess dietary sugar and alcohol can cause a B_2 deficiency. We must eat foods containing this vitamin regularly, for little is stored in the body.

Selected Sources of Vitamin B_2

Food	Serving Size	Vitamin B_2 (mg)
Liver	3 oz, braised	3.5
Turkey heart	1 c, cooked	1.3
Chicken	½, roasted	.5
Gefilte fish	3 oz	.3
Sardines, canned	3 oz	.3
Sweet potato	½ peeled, mashed	.2
Spinach	½ c raw, chopped	.1
Turnip greens	½ c chopped cooked	.1

Vitamin B_6

Like other vitamins, B_6 is really a "mini-family" of related substances. Three substances, pyridoxine, pyridoxal, and pyridoxamine, are collectively called vitamin B_6.

Vitamin B_6's Duties: B_6 is involved with a variety of body functions. Its most important tasks have to do with protein; helping to manufacture amino acids from carbohydrates, converting one amino acid to another, and transforming the amino acid tryptophan to the vitamin niacin. B_6 plays an important role in the production of hormones, neurotransmitters, and the hemoglobin in the red blood cells that holds oxygen. B_6 also aids in the extraction of energy from carbohydrates, fats and proteins.

Studies have shown that B_6 can be an effective treatment for certain cases of asthma, mood and sleep disorders, carpal tunnel syndrome, and premenstrual syndrome. The Physician's Health Study found that low levels of B_6 and folic acid are associated with heart disease. Other studies have revealed that low levels of B_6 are associated with weakened immune systems.

Deficiency Signs and Symptoms: Because the vitamin is involved in so many different metabolic systems, the symptoms of a B_6 deficiency are vague and affect many different parts of the body. Deficiency symptoms include problems with the immune system, nervousness, weakness, loss of appetite and weight, abnormal heart rhythms, insomnia, anemia, inflammation of the nerves, and lethargy. The elderly, who may have age-related absorption difficulties, are often deficient in the vitamin, despite eating adequate amounts of foods containing the B_6. The Second National U.S. Health and Nutrition Examination Survey found that 90 percent of females, and 71 percent of males, were consuming less than the RDA for this vitamin.

Where to Find It and Other Vital Information: Meat, poultry, fish, soybeans, dried beans, peas, and other protein-rich foods are good sources of vitamin B_6. This vitamin is also found in cabbage, cauliflower, potatoes, whole-grain breads, and bananas. Freezing vegetables and exposing foods to light lowers their B_6 content. We must eat foods containing this vitamin regularly, for little is stored in the body.

Selected Sources of Vitamin B_6

Food	Serving Size	Vitamin B_6 (mg)
Avocado, Florida	1 medium	.9
Beef liver	3 oz, braised	.8
Turkey, light meat	1 cup, roasted	.8
Banana	1 medium	.7
Chicken	½ chicken, roasted	.7
Salmon, smoked	3 oz	.6
Sea bass	3 oz, cooked	.4
Mackerel	3 oz, cooked	.4
Snapper	3 oz, cooked	.4
Rainbow trout	3 oz, cooked	.4
Wheat germ	¼ c, toasted	.3
Corn	½ c	.2
Walnuts	1 oz	.2
Yogurt, nonfat	1 c	.1

Vitamin B$_{12}$
(Also known as cobalamin and cyanocobalamin)

The B$_{12}$ story begins with a fatal disease which was given the name "pernicious anemia" in the 1800s. Doctors later discovered that eating a pound of raw liver a day cured the disease. It wasn't until 1940, however, that researchers isolated the factor in liver that cured this anemia, and named it "vitamin B$_{12}$."

Vitamin B$_{12}$'s Duties: The body uses vitamin B$_{12}$ to metabolize carbohydrates, fat, and protein; to produce acids; to synthesize DNA; and to keep the nervous and immune systems healthy. B$_{12}$ aids in the production and growth of red blood cells in the bone marrow, and their release into the circulatory system when they are mature.

Deficiency Signs and Symptoms: B$_{12}$ is a vital part of the red blood cell's life cycle. That's why a deficiency of this vitamin leads to an anemia deadly enough to be called "pernicious." Other deficiency symptoms include dizziness, forgetfulness, weakness, an enlargement of the spleen, headaches, heart palpitations, constipation, bruising, immune-system weakness, and problems with blood-clotting mechanisms. The symptoms of a B$_{12}$ deficiency are similar to those of diabetic neuropathy (nerve damage caused by diabetes), leading researchers to wonder if B$_{12}$ isn't also implicated in diabetes.

Where to Find It and Other Vital Information: Vitamin B$_{12}$ is only found in meat, poultry, milk, and other foods of animal origin—there is no B$_{12}$ in vegetables, fruits, or other foods that grow in or above the ground. The only non-animal foods that have B$_{12}$ are those that have been fermented by B$_{12}$-producing bacteria, such as miso. Excessive boiling and exposure to light can lower the B$_{12}$ content of foods. We must eat foods containing this vitamin regularly, for little is stored in the body.

Selected Sources of Vitamin B₁₂

Food	Serving Size	Vitamin B_{12} (mcg)
Turkey liver	1 c cooked	66.5
Clams	3 oz, steamed	43.4
Mussels in tomato sauce	¾ c, cooked	32.4
Oysters, smoked	3 oz	25
Salmon, smoked	3 oz	6
Tuna	3 oz, broiled	3
Salmon, fresh	3 oz, broiled	2
Milk, skim	1 c	1

Vitamin C
(Also known as ascorbic acid)

Perhaps the most famous of the vitamins, C has been embroiled in controversy ever since double-Nobel-prize–winning scientist Linus Pauling announced that it could cure the common cold.

Vitamin C's Duties: Vitamin C is vital for a healthy immune system. It also helps to protect the body from oxidation, helps to regulate cholesterol levels, and encourages the absorption of iron from the food we eat. Perhaps its most important function has to do with helping to manufacture and maintain collagen, a protein that serves as a "cement" between cells and the basis for connective tissue. Collagen is everywhere in the body, including the bones, teeth, tendons, skin, and the blood vessels.

A great deal of study suggests that vitamin C can help asthmatics breathe easier; can speed up recovery from pneumonia, mononucleosis, hepatitis, and other viral infections; can strengthen the immune system by stimulating T-cells, B-cells, and the "cell eaters" (macrophages) that ingest and destroy bacteria, viruses, and other invaders; can protect the heart by regulating the liver's production of cholesterol and by helping to remove cholesterol from artery walls; and can aid in the fight against cancer through its antioxidant properties.

During the mid-1980s, researchers discovered a novel use for vitamin C—weight loss. Acting on the theory that vitamin C would rev up the sodium pump found in the body's cells, thus forcing the cells to burn more energy, they gave supplemental vitamin C to obese volunteers. In one such study, 38 women whose weights averaged 50 percent over the ideal, and who had not succeeded on diets, were given either 3 grams of vitamin C or a placebo daily, and told to eat whatever they desired. Six weeks later, the vitamin C takers had lost twice as much weight as those on the placebo.

Deficiency Signs and Symptoms: A deficiency of C can cause damage to blood vessels, swelling and tenderness of the joints, bone aches, muscle cramps, poor healing of wounds, the breakdown of old scars, irritability, bleeding and inflammation of the gums, bruising, hemorrhages (bleeding) under the skin, shortness of breath, and other problems. A serious deficiency leads to scurvy. It's felt that up to 50 percent of American women take in less than the RDA for C daily. The elderly, men living alone, and alcoholics are at risk for developing deficiencies.

Where to Find It and Other Vital Information: The best sources of vitamin C are fresh vegetables and fruits, such as sweet red peppers, snow peas, strawberries, Brussels sprouts, tangerines, papaya, grapefruit, broccoli, and tomatoes. Vitamin C may be lost from food if the food is bruised, overwashed, overcooked, reheated, processed, or exposed to the air. Both alcohol and stress increase the need for the vitamin. We must eat foods containing this vitamin regularly, for little is stored in the body.

Selected Sources of Vitamin C

Food	Serving Size	Vitamin C (mg)
Papaya	1 medium	188
Guava	1 raw	165
Peppers, red	1 raw	141
Cantaloupe	½	113
Black currants	½ c	101
Peppers, sweet green	1 raw	97
Kiwi	1 raw	75
Orange	1	70
Broccoli	½ c, chopped, cooked	49
Cauliflower	½ c, pieces, cooked	34
Asparagus	½ c, cooked	24

Vitamin D

Sometimes called the "sunshine vitamin," vitamin D can be made by the human body—but only with exposure to sunlight.

Vitamin D's Duties: Vitamin D is actually a group of three related compounds (D_1, D_2, D_3) that help to regulate the absorption and use of calcium and phosphorus. Thus, vitamin D plays a major role in the strength and health of bones and teeth. The vitamin is also important for the health of nerve cells and muscles.

Deficiency Signs and Symptoms: A deficiency can lead to tooth decay and disorders of the nervous system. In children, the classic D deficiency disease is rickets, often characterized by bowed legs that have buckled under the strain of trying to support the body, and by weak, malformed bones elsewhere in the body. In adults, a severe deficiency leads to osteomalacia, the adult form of rickets. Osteomalacia is most often seen in women whose calcium stores have been depleted by repeated pregnancies and a poor diet, and/or who almost completely cover their bodies, including their faces, hands, arms, and legs, with clothing, preventing the sunlight from touching their skin. It may also be found among night workers and elderly shut-ins who have little exposure to the sun (and often a poor diet).

Where to Find It and Other Vital Information: The best food source of vitamin D is vitamin D–fortified milk. Cod liver oil and other fish oils are also good sources. Herring, salmon, sardines, liver, cream, and egg yolk have variable amounts of this vitamin. Although fortified milk is a good source of D, dairy products such as cheese are not, for they are rarely made with fortified milk.

Vitamin E
(Also known as tocopherol)

First identified as the substance from food that, if absent, made laboratory rats infertile, vitamin E was given the scientific name of tocopherol, which means "to bring forth children." Today, however, E is receiving much more attention for its antioxidant properties than for its ability to ensure procreation.

"Vitamin E" is actually a family of eight different naturally occurring substances, half of which belong to the tocopherol family and half of which are tocotrienols. Alpha tocopherol is the most active and common form of E.

Vitamin E's Duties: Vitamin E is an antioxidant which guards against oxidation damage. Its duties include protecting the eyes, skin, liver, muscles, and breast tissue; preventing pollution damage to the mouth and lungs; and preventing damage to red blood cells. (Vitamin E is often added to skin-care preparations for its protective antioxidant effects.)

A large number of studies have suggested that the antioxidant E is a potent weapon in the fight against cancer and heart disease, a shield against the ravages of aging, an immune system booster, and an effective treatment for osteoarthritis.

Deficiency Signs and Symptoms: A deficiency of vitamin E can lead to disorders of the nervous system, premature aging of the skin, infertility, and destruction of red blood cells.

Where to Find It and Other Vital Information: Fortunately, vitamin E is found in a great many foods, including wheat germ oil, green leafy vegetables, broccoli, Brussels sprouts, green beans, nuts, and seeds. Meat and other foods of animal origin are generally not very good sources of E.

This fat-soluble vitamin is stored in the body. Large doses of E appear to be harmless, although they may cause slower clotting of the blood in certain individuals by reducing the level of clotting factors associated with vitamin K.

Vitamin K

A relatively "unknown" vitamin, K is a family of three related substances: K_1 occurs naturally in green plants, K_2 is formed by bacteria in the intestinal tract, and K_3 is a very potent, synthetic version of the vitamin.

Vitamin K's Duties: Vitamin K's primary function is to help regulate blood clotting. Too little K can lead to abnormally slow clotting. The vitamin may also play a role in slowing the growth of cancers of the stomach, bladder, liver, kidney, breast, ovary, and colon.

Deficiency Signs and Symptoms: Deficiencies of vitamin K are rare. They do occur in some newborns, because it may be a few days or weeks before their intestinal bacteria begin making sufficient amounts of the vitamin. Newborns are often given injections of K. Mothers-to-be may be given K supplements to ensure that enough of the vitamin gets to the almost-born child, and that there will be sufficient K in the breast milk.

In adults, deficiencies only occur under special circumstances, such as if one is taking antibiotics that interfere with intestinal bacteria, or other medicines that interfere with the absorption or use of K. Minor deficiencies may be common among pregnant women.

Where to Find It: Vitamin K is found in broccoli, Romaine lettuce, cabbage, and other green or leafy vegetables, as well as in liver, egg yolk and other foods.

OTHER VITAMIN-LIKE SUBSTANCES

In addition to the vitamins, several other substances in food are necessary for good health and growth.

Bioflavonoids (Flavonoids): Originally called "vitamin P," this group of over 200 plant pigments has powerful antioxidant properties. Individual bioflavonoids are helpful in treating fragile capillaries, bleeding gums, and allergic inflammation. Currently, studies are being done to find out if bioflavonoids are effective in fighting viruses.

Some of the many bioflavonoids are hesperidin, rutin, queretin and catechin. Bioflavonoids are found in the outer layers, skin and peels of vegetables and fruits, in leafy vegetables, coffee, tea and wine.

Choline: Although not considered a vitamin, choline is an essential nutrient with important functions in the body. The body can manufacture choline with the aid of folic acid, vitamin B_{12}, and an amino acid called methionine. The body's own production of choline is usually too low to meet daily requirements, so additional choline is needed from the diet.

Choline helps to clear fat from the liver, build cell walls, and keep the brain and nerves running smoothly. Choline is transformed into a neurotransmitter called acetylcholine in the brain. In this form, it plays an important role in keeping the memory sharp. Researchers are investigating a possible link between choline, memory and Alzheimer's disease.

Clinical deficiencies of choline are not known to occur in humans, except under laboratory conditions. Healthy volunteers given a choline-poor diet have suffered from liver dysfunction. The best food source of choline is egg yolk. Liver, kidney, brain, yeast, soybeans, green peas, and peanuts also contain choline.

Inositol: Although generally recognized as a vitamin, inositol can be made by both the body and intestinal bacteria. It is not known, however, if the average person makes enough inositol to meet daily requirements, or whether additional inositol is required from the diet.

Inositol is found throughout the body, in the brain, nerves, heart, reproductive system, muscles, and bones. It is a part of cell walls, and plays a role in the transmission of nerve signals and the production of certain enzymes. It also helps to prevent the buildup of fats in the liver and other organs.

Inositol deficiencies do not occur because the substance is found in so many foods. In animals, lack of inositol leads to the accumulation of fat in the liver, and problems with the nerve and intestines. Inositol is found in vegetables, fruits, grains, nuts, organ meats and many other foods. Excessive amounts of inositol are not known to have any damaging effects upon the body.

Lipoic Acid: Although lipoic acid is not a vitamin, it works with several of the B vitamins in order to break down fat, protein and carbohydrates for energy. Lipoic acid is found in liver and in brewer's yeast. It is not known how much lipoic acid one needs every day, exactly what happens if one is lacking lipoic acid, or if an excess is toxic.

Ubiquinone (Coenzyme Q$_{10}$): Ubiquinone is actually a family of related substances known as the ubiquinones. The name comes from the fact that the substance is ubiquitous (found almost everywhere) in both foods and in the body. Produced by the body, ubiquinone helps the body convert carbohydrates into energy.

Cardiologists have been using ubiquinone to strengthen the heartbeat in patients with weak hearts for many years. Studies suggest that the vitamin-like substance may also strengthen the immune system, help the body resist the ravages of aging, assist in keeping blood pressure and weight in check, and may even prove to be useful in the treatment of certain cancers.

It is not known how much ubiquinone one needs every day, what the deficiency symptoms might be, or if an excess is harmful.

THE VITAMIN TEAM

Although we think of the vitamins individually, they are more like a team of nutrients working together to promote growth and health. We need large amounts of some vitamins and small amounts of others, and some have more "prestigious" jobs than the others, but all the vitamins and minerals must work together if we are to remain healthy. For example:

- Vitamin B$_2$ activates B$_6$.
- Vitamins B$_1$, B$_2$, B$_6$, and B$_{12}$ work together to extract energy from carbohydrates, protein, and fat. A deficiency of any one of them can hamper the others.

- Proper amounts of B_6 are required to absorb B_{12} from food.
- The body needs pantothenic acid in order to manufacture vitamin D.
- Vitamin E's antioxidant abilities are enhanced by the presence of the mineral selenium.
- The body needs zinc in order to transport and use vitamin A.
- Vitamin D is required for the absorption and use of calcium and phosphorus.
- More iron is absorbed from food if the meal also contains vitamin C.

However, the vitamin team must be kept in balance. Too much of a good thing can be harmful. For example:

- Excessive E can interfere with vitamin K's coagulant duties.
- Long-term, excessive intake of an amino acid called leucine can lead to a deficiency of tryptophan. And since the body converts some tryptophan to niacin, too much leucine can also lead to a niacin deficiency.

Balance is the key to good nutrient teamwork, which is why it's important not to overlook or to overemphasize nutrients. The B vitamins, for example, work together to convert food into energy. Taking massive doses of any one of them probably won't make you more energetic—making sure that you're getting good amounts of all of them is a better approach.

How can you ensure that your vitamin team is balanced? No single food contains all the nutrients and phytochemicals needed for vibrant health, so the best approach is to eat a wide variety of foods, with special emphasis on fresh vegetables and fruits, plus whole grains. The Food & Nutrition Board, which sets the RDAs, suggests eating 5 or more servings of vegetables and fruits every day, especially green and yellow vegetables and citrus fruits; 6 or more daily servings of peas, beans, breads, and other foods high in complex carbohydrates; and 6 ounces or less of lean meat per day; and limiting your consumption of fats, fried foods, fatty foods, oils and egg yolks. (An average serving is ½ cup of cooked or one cup of raw fruits and vegetables, ½ cup of cooked or dry cereal, one slice of bread, 1 muffin or roll, or 1 medium piece of fruit.)

Your physician or health adviser can help you analyze your nutrient intake, and make any necessary recommendations for changing your diet or taking supplements. Many health professionals, including dietitians and some chiropractors, can analyze your diet to determine how much of each nutrient you are eating. Physicians can perform blood tests to check the nutrient levels in your blood. Newer tests offered by laboratories such as Spectro Cell in Houston can actually determine how well your body utilizes the nutrients in the blood.

THE RECOMMENDED DAILY ALLOWANCES FOR VITAMINS

To help people determine how much of the essential nutrients are needed for good health and growth, the National Academy of Sciences' Food & Nutrition Board has established Recommended Daily Allowances (RDAs) for several essential nutrients. Figure 2.1 on pages 44–45 shows the RDAs for vitamins.

In addition, the Food & Nutrition Board has a devised a table of "safe and adequate daily dietary intakes" for biotin and pantothenic acid. The intake ranges are:

Figure 2.2. Safe and Adequate Ranges For Vitamins

Estimated Safe and Adequate Daily Dietary Intakes
of Selected Vitamins

Category	Age (years)	Biotin (mcg)	Pantothenic Acid (mg)
Infants	0–0.5	10	2
	0.5–1	15	3
Children	1–3	20	3
and adolescents	4–6	25	3–4
	7–10	30	4–5
	11+	30–100	4–7
Adults	18+	30–100	4–7

The RDAs and the "safe and adequate daily dietary intakes" are only guidelines, estimates of a healthy person's needs. Unfortunately, the RDAs are set too low. They are sufficient to stave off disease, but do not promote optimal health.

Figure 2.1. RDA for Vitamins

Food & Nutrition Board, National Academy of Sciences—National Research Council
Recommended Dietary Allowances. Revised 1989.

Vitamins

	Age	A (RE)[1]	B$_1$ (mg)	B$_2$ (mg)	B$_6$ (mg)	B$_{12}$ (mcg)	C (mg)	D (mcg)	E (mg)	K (mcg)	Niacin (mg)	Folate (mcg)
Infants	0.0–0.5	375	0.3	0.4	0.3	0.3	30	7.5	3	5	5	25
	0.5–1.0	375	0.4	0.5	0.6	0.5	35	10	4	10	6	35
Children	1–3	400	0.7	0.8	1.0	0.7	40	10	6	15	9	50
	4–6	500	0.9	1.1	1.1	1.0	45	10	7	20	12	75
	7–10	700	1.0	1.2	1.4	1.4	45	10	7	30	13	100
Males	11–14	1,000	1.3	1.5	1.7	2.0	50	10	10	45	17	150
	15–18	1,000	1.5	1.8	2.0	2.0	60	10	10	65	20	200
	19–24	1,000	1.5	1.7	2.0	2.0	60	10	10	70	19	200
	25–50	1,000	1.5	1.7	2.0	2.0	60	5	10	80	19	200
	51+	1,000	1.2	1.4	2.0	2.0	60	5	10	80	15	200

Females												
	11–14	800	1.1	1.3	1.4	2.0	50	10	8	45	15	150
	15–18	800	1.1	1.3	1.5	2.0	60	10	8	55	15	180
	19–24	800	1.1	1.3	1.6	2.0	60	10	8	60	15	180
	25–50	800	1.1	1.3	1.6	2.0	60	5	8	65	15	180
	51+	800	1.0	1.2	1.6	2.0	60	5	8	65	13	180
Pregnant		800	1.5	1.6	2.2	2.2	70	10	10	65	17	400
Lactating[2]		1,300	1.6	1.8	2.1	2.6	95	10	12	65	20	280

[1]RE = retinal equivalents, a measure of vitamin A activity. 1 RE = 33.3 IU (international units) of vitamin A or 10 IU of beta carotene.

[2]Although the RDAs are given separately for the first and second six months of lactation, I've included only the figures for the first six months, which are slightly higher in a few categories.

Caution: It *is* possible to get too much of a good thing. Although a lack of vitamins is the greater problem, vitamin excess can also be harmful. Here are some of the signs and symptoms of vitamin overdose:

Vitamin A: Vitamin A is safe if taken in normal amounts. If you take supplements containing 50,000 or more International Units (IU) per day for several months or years, you may develop nausea, joint pain, irritability, drowsiness, skin problems, enlargement of the spleen and liver, and other problems. The latest research indicates that pregnant women should take no more than 5,000 IU of vitamin A per day, if any at all, because larger doses may cause birth defects.

Beta-carotene: No overdose symptoms are known, for the body apparently only converts as much beta-carotene to vitamin A as is necessary, allowing the rest to be excreted in the urine.

Biotin: This vitamin is nontoxic.

Folic Acid: Even when taken in doses 1,000 times the RDA, folic acid has no known toxic effects.

Niacin: Very large doses (1,000 mg or more) of supplemental niacin can cause flushing of the skin, headaches, and other transient problems. Because folic acid works with B_{12}, too much folic acid could "hide" a B_{12} deficiency, allowing the deficiency to continue until irreversible nerve damage has been done.

Pantothenic Acid: Taking large amounts may cause diarrhea.

Vitamin B_1: Very little B_1 is stored in the body, so it is unlikely that enough will build up to be harmful. It appears that one can take up to 300 mg of B_1 per day, many times the RDA, without suffering any adverse effects.

Vitamin B_2: This vitamin has no known toxic effects.

Vitamin B_6: Studies have shown that injecting large doses (30 or more times greater than the RDA) of B_6 can cause sleepiness. Doses 100 or more times greater than the RDA can cause poor coordination, degeneration of the nerve tissue and other problems.

Vitamin B_{12}: This vitamin is nontoxic.

Vitamin C: Excess vitamin C is excreted in the urine. However, large amounts of the vitamin may interfere with test results for diabetes and hemoglobin, and may cause diarrhea, nausea, and other stomach problems. Those who have been taking large doses of C but then stop may suffer from "rebound scurvy" caused by the body's habituation to the large amounts of C. Some studies have found that large amounts of the vitamin may encourage the formation of kidney stones.

Vitamin D: This fat-soluble vitamin is stored in the body, so levels can climb too high. Symptoms of a D-overdose include dermatitis, headaches, loss of appetite, diarrhea, irreversible damage to the heart and kidney, excessive calcification of the bones, and mental retardation.

Vitamin E: Vitamin E appears to be very safe, although taking large doses may slow blood-clotting time by interfering with vitamin K. This is most likely to happen to people taking anticoagulation medicines for heart problems, or those with liver disease, which lowers vitamin K levels in the body.

Vitamin K: Infants given large doses of the synthetic K suffer from brain damage, and animals given the synthetic vitamin develop anemia. For this reason, Vitamin K supplements are only available by prescription. The natural form found in foods is very safe.

Caution: Taking vitamin supplements might *be dangerous if you are also taking medications. For example, vitamin C may interfere with medicines such as Coumadin™, which are used to thin the blood—and vitamin K definitely counteracts Coumadin™. If you are taking Accutane™ for acne, don't take supplemental vitamin A because the medicine is a relative of the vitamin, and taking the two together may lead to toxicity. Taking extra folic acid and vitamin B_6 may interfere with drugs used for convulsions, possibly triggering a seizure. And you should not take extra B_6 if you have Parkinson's disease and are taking an L-dopa-type drug such as Larodopa™ or Dopar™. These are just some of the potential supplement-drug interactions. Be sure to tell your physician if you are taking any vitamins or other supplements.*

CHAPTER 3

What Minerals Do for You

The minerals we need to sustain health and life are common substances such as calcium, potassium, silicon, and tin. The 22 essential minerals and the many other minerals found in the average human account for between 4 and 5 percent of body weight (meaning that there are about 7 pounds of minerals inside the body of a 150-pound person).

The essential minerals are divided into two groups, according to how much of each is found in the body. The major minerals are present in larger amounts (more than 0.005 percent of body weight), while the trace minerals are present in smaller amounts. Think of the distinction this way: If there is more than a teaspoon's worth of a mineral in the body, it's a major mineral; if less, it's a trace mineral.

The major minerals are calcium, chloride, magnesium, phosphorus, potassium, sodium, and sulfur.

The trace minerals are chromium, cobalt, copper, fluoride, iodine, iron, manganese, molybdenum, nickel, selenium, silicon, tin, and zinc.

Major and trace minerals are equally essential; some are simply needed in larger quantities than others. Other nonessential minerals found in the body include arsenic, boron, barium, cadmium, and mercury. Their roles in health and disease are not yet well understood, although we know that large doses of minerals such as arsenic and mercury can be toxic. Let's take a look at the essential major and trace minerals, then at the others.

ESSENTIAL MAJOR AND TRACE MINERALS

Calcium

Calcium contributes 2 ½ to 3 pounds to the average healthy man's weight, and accounts for approximately 2 pounds of the average healthy woman's weight. Just about all of the calcium in the human body is locked up in the bones and teeth, with only about 1 percent circulating in the blood and other body fluids, or in the cells.

Calcium's Duties: Calcium's best-known job is keeping the bones and teeth strong. Some of the calcium in bones is more or less permanent, while another portion is "stored" there in case the amount of calcium in the blood falls too low. If that happens, calcium is "withdrawn" from this "bone-bank" and used for other body functions. Too many "withdrawals" can damage the bones in the long run.

Calcium also plays a major role in maintaining blood pressure at the proper level. The first National Health & Nutrition Examination Survey found that low calcium levels are linked to high blood pressure. In fact, this and other studies suggest that, for heart patients, getting enough calcium may be even more important than keeping sodium (salt) levels down.

Calcium is also necessary in order for the blood to clot, for the nerves to transmit signals, for the muscles to contract, and for various enzyme systems to function. Calcium helps to prevent muscle cramps, irregular heartbeat, and skin problems, as well as certain types of insomnia, depression, delusions, and cognitive impairment.

Deficiency Signs and Symptoms: A lack of calcium may cause tetany (pain and spastic contractions of the muscles), high blood pressure, osteoporosis ("thin bones") in adults and rickets in children. Most people, especially adult women, pregnant women, and the elderly, are not getting enough calcium.

Where to Find It and Other Vital Information: Milk, cheese, tofu, dried figs, yogurt, and sardines (with bones) are good sources of calcium.

Only 10 to 40 percent of the calcium in foods is actually

absorbed into the body—and that figure may be lower in post-menopausal women. The body's ability to absorb calcium can be hindered by the oxalates and phytates found in spinach and other foods, by a lack of vitamin D in the diet, by excess dietary fat, stress, certain drugs (such as the antibiotic tetracycline and diuretics that flush water from the body), and other factors.

Selected Sources of Calcium

Food	Serving Size	Calcium (mg)
Milk, nonfat	1 c	302
Milk, low-fat	1 c	300
Milk, whole	1 c	291
Buttermilk	1 c	285
Figs, dried	10 (6.6 oz)	269
Swiss cheese	1 oz	219
Oysters, smoked	3 oz	130
Spinach	½ c, cooked	122
Tofu (bean curd)	½ c	118
Broccoli	½ c, chopped, cooked	89
Almonds, dry-roasted	1 oz	80
Papaya	1 medium	72
Raisins, seedless	1 c	71
Barley, pearled	1 c, dry	68
Orange	1	52
Okra	½ c, sliced, cooked	50

Chloride

Chloride, which is found in the body's fluids, works closely with sodium and potassium to maintain the proper distribution of water throughout the body, to keep the acid-base balance at the proper level, and to help muscles contract at the right times. Most of the body's chloride is found in the fluids which bathe body cells.

Chloride's Duties: As part of the stomach's acids, chloride plays a role in digesting food. Working with sodium and potassium, chloride helps to ensure that fluids are properly balanced and distributed throughout the body. These three minerals also ensure that the muscles and nervous system function properly.

Deficiency Signs and Symptoms: Chloride deficiency may lead to diarrhea, muscle weakness, lethargy, vomiting, and other problems, including coma. Excessive vomiting, such as the kind that occurs with bulimia, may lead to a chloride deficiency.

Where to Find It: Chloride is found in vegetables, grains, fruits, meat, poultry, and dairy products. The greatest amount is found in table salt, but there is plenty of chloride in other foods. You don't have to add salt just to get chloride.

Chromium

Infants have the greatest concentrations of chromium, with amounts falling as one ages. The muscles, brain, adrenal glands and your body's fat all contain chromium.

Chromium's Duties: Chromium's main role is helping the body to utilize glucose (sugar). As a part of the glucose tolerance factor (GTF), chromium regulates the levels of glucose in the blood, and helps to move the sugar into the cells when appropriate. That's why a diet low in chromium can cause the appearance of diabetes-like symptoms, such as increased blood sugar, glucose intolerance, and numbness and tingling of the fingers and toes. Chromium may also play a role in helping to keep cholesterol under control.

Deficiency Signs and Symptoms: Elevated cholesterol, glucose intolerance, impaired growth, fatigue, and anxiety have all been associated with a deficiency of chromium.

Up to 90 percent of all Americans may be eating diets low in chromium. Small but significant deficiencies of chromium are common among people eating the standard American diet, thanks to the large amounts of sugars and refined foods consumed.

Where to Find It: Chromium is found in brewer's yeast, oysters, liver, and potatoes (with the skins), as well as in seafood, cheeses, meats, and whole grains.

Cobalt

The human body contains only very small amounts of cobalt. This mineral is the only one of the essential elements that is actually a part of a vitamin (B_{12}).

Cobalt's Duties: Without cobalt, there can be no vitamin B_{12}. As part of B_{12}, cobalt helps the body metabolize carbohydrates, fat, and protein; produce amino acids; synthesize DNA; and keep the nervous and immune systems healthy. Vitamin B_{12} is responsible for the proper functioning of all body cells, as well as for the manufacture and growth of red blood cells.

Deficiency Signs and Symptoms: A lack of cobalt, which is equivalent to a deficiency of vitamin B_{12}, can lead to pernicious anemia and many other problems. (See the discussion of B_{12} on page 34.)

Where to Find It: Although fruits, vegetables, and many other foods contain cobalt, the body prefers cobalt which is already incorporated into vitamin B_{12}. So when looking for foods containing cobalt, think of B_{12} foods such as organ and muscle meats. Because meat is the best source of cobalt/vitamin B_{12}, strict vegetarians may be at risk of deficiency.

Copper

Although it is concentrated in the heart, liver, brain, and kidneys, copper is found throughout the body. In a general sense, the body treats copper much as it does iron, metabolizing them in the same way.

Copper's Duties: As a part of many enzyme systems, copper plays a role in the proper growth and/or maintenance of the heart, bones, nerves, brain, and red blood cells. Copper helps the body derive energy from protein, carbohydrates, and fat, and assists in the manufacture of the hormone-like prostaglandins. The prostaglandins, in turn, regulate the blood pressure and heartbeat, and contribute to the healing of wounds.

New evidence suggests that copper plays a role in pain perception by ensuring that there are enough enkephalins to control pain. (Enkephalins are endorphins, hormones made by the body to help regulate pain by blocking the transmission of certain pain signals through the nervous system.)

As part of superoxide dismutase (SOD), an enzyme that

protects body cells from oxidation damage, copper may play a role in fighting cancer and heart disease, and may help the body to resist the ravages of aging. Copper may also be important to strong bones. Epidemiological studies have linked the typical Western low-copper diet to the high rates of osteoporosis in the Western world.

Deficiency Signs and Symptoms: Copper deficiency may lead to heart problems, elevated blood pressure, damage to the blood vessels and skin, bone deformities, depression, fatigue, weakness, anemia, diarrhea, scoliosis, breathing difficulties, infections, and blood disorders.

Where to Find It: Whole-grain cereals and breads, nuts, organ meats, dark green, leafy vegetables, poultry, peas, and beans all contain copper.

Fluoride

Although there is less than an ounce of fluoride in the typical adult body, this mineral plays an important role in maintaining healthy teeth and bones.

Fluoride's Duties: Fluoride's main function is to guard against tooth decay. The numbers of new cavities have decreased since communities began fluoridating their water supplies. (Too much fluoride, however, can cause the teeth to mottle.) Fluoride works best while the teeth are still growing, so it's wise to start using fluoridated water and toothpaste early. Fluoride also helps to strengthen the bones, making them more resistant to osteoporosis. As with the teeth, however, too much fluoride may be harmful, possibly increasing the risk of hairline fractures.

Deficiency Signs and Symptoms: Lack of fluoride in drinking water is linked to an increased incidence of tooth decay.

Where to Find It: The primary source of dietary fluoride is fluoridated drinking water. Fish is also a good source of the mineral.

Iodine

The greatest concentration of iodine is found in the thyroid gland, which is wrapped around the trachea. The addition of iodine to salt solved the once-serious goiter problem in several regions of the United States.

Iodine's Duties: Iodine is necessary to make the thyroid hormone thyroxine, which regulates growth, reproduction, neuromuscular function, the growth of the hair and skin, energy transformation, and the metabolic rate. Thyroxin helps to control body weight by controlling the way in which the body uses energy.

Deficiency Signs and Symptoms: A lack of iodine can lead to simple or endemic goiter. When the body runs low of iodine and cannot manufacture enough thyroid hormones, the thyroid gland tries to compensate by swelling in size. The result is a large lump at the front of the neck called a goiter. Goiter, which is easily treated by increasing the amount of iodine in the diet, is more common in areas where the soil is poor in iodine, and the foods grown in these soils are also deficient. It is so common in some countries that it is considered a "normal" development rather than an illness.

Goiter can also be caused by eating foods containing substances that naturally inhibit the thyroid gland. These foods include raw mustard seeds, turnips, peanuts, cauliflower, and rutabagas. Certain drugs, such as thiouracil, can also cause goiter.

Where to Find It: Iodine is found in variable amounts in foods, depending on the amount of iodine in the soil where the food was grown. The amount of iodine in drinking water also varies. The most consistent source of iodine is iodized salt.

Iron

Most of the iron in the human body (some 70 percent) is used to hold oxygen in the red blood cells as the cells move to the far reaches of the body. About one-fifth of the body's iron is stored in organs such as the liver and the spleen, with the remainder being found in the muscles, body cells, and fluids.

Iron's Duties: Iron's primary duty is to make up part of the hemoglobin molecule found in red blood cells. As the red cells pass through the lungs, the hemoglobin binds to fresh oxygen. Oxygen is released by the red blood cells at the appropriate junctures in the blood vessels. Iron also increases the resistance to disease by strengthening the immune system.

Deficiency Signs and Symptoms: Lack of iron may lead to ane-mia, heart disease, deterioration of mental skills, constipation, digestive problems, dizziness, fragile bones, fatigue, head-aches, and other problems.

Iron deficiency is the most prevalent deficiency among American children, and is common in adolescents. The RDA for iron is higher for girls and women between the ages of 11 and 50 than it is for men because women lose iron during menstruation.

Where to Find It and Other Vital Information: Organ meats, dark green, leafy vegetables, fish, poultry, peas, and beans are all good sources of iron. Only 10 to 30 percent of the iron in foods is absorbed. Absorption can be hindered by gastrointes-tinal disease, infections, as well as by the phosphate, phytate and oxalates in foods. Absorption is aided by vitamin C, cal-cium and stomach acids.

Selected Sources of Iron

Food	Serving Size	Iron (mg)
Calf's liver	3½ oz, cooked	14.0
Oysters, smoked	3 oz	8.0
Pumpkin seeds	1 oz	4.0
Beet greens	3½ oz, raw	3.2
Lentils	½ c, cooked	2.1
Brewer's yeast	1 T	1.0

Magnesium

Over half of the body's magnesium is found in the bones, with the rest being distributed among the body fluids and soft tissues (including the heart). Sometimes called "calcium's op-posite," magnesium helps to balance some of calcium's ef-fects. For example, while we need calcium to contract smooth muscles, magnesium helps those muscles relax.

Magnesium's Duties: Calcium, which makes muscles con-tract, can cause the smooth muscles surrounding the blood vessels in the heart to constrict. Squeezing down on the vital blood vessels, the muscles may reduce blood flow, causing chest pain and possibly contributing to a heart attack. Mag-nesium acts in opposition to calcium, helping to keep the blood flowing by relaxing the smooth muscles wrapped around the blood vessels.

Magnesium is also needed for protein synthesis, to remove certain toxic substances from the body, to keep the nervous system functioning, and to convert fat, carbohydrates, and protein into energy.

Magnesium can improve the odds of surviving a heart attack, keep the blood from clotting unnecessarily, lessen the symptoms of premenstrual syndrome in many women, and help certain kinds of diabetics to keep their blood pressure in check. Magnesium may also lower the bad LDL cholesterol, while increasing the beneficial HDL cholesterol.

Deficiency Signs and Symptoms: A lack of magnesium may produce a variety of symptoms, including irregular heartbeat, loss of appetite, muscle spasms and weakness, and poor coordination.

Although serious deficiencies of magnesium are rare, it is felt that marginal shortcomings are common, with perhaps as few as 25 percent of all Americans taking in the RDA for this mineral. The elderly, pregnant women, and patients hospitalized for gastrointestinal disorders such as prolonged diarrhea or vomiting are more likely to have a magnesium deficiency.

Where to Find It: Nuts, whole-grain breads, peas, beans, and dark green, leafy vegetables are good sources of magnesium.

Selected Sources of Magnesium

Food	Serving Size	Magnesium (mg)
Pumpkin kernels, roasted	1 oz	152
All-bran cereal	⅓ c	106
Avocado	1	104
Tofu (bean curd)	½ c	94
Almonds, dry-roasted	1 oz	86
Filberts, dried	1 oz	81
Spinach	½ c, cooked	79
Swiss chard	½ c, chopped, cooked	76
Lima beans	½ c, raw	63
Noodles, whole-wheat	1 c, cooked	59

Manganese

Weighing in at less than an ounce, the body's stores of manganese are primarily located in the liver, pituitary gland, bones, and pancreas. Compared to the other minerals, we know relatively little about manganese. In fact, the first case of manganese deficiency was not recognized until the early 1970s.

Manganese's Duties: Acting as an enzyme, manganese is involved in many metabolic reactions. It plays a role in the synthesis of proteins, bones and cholesterol, helps the body to digest proteins, and it is necessary for blood clotting.

Deficiency Signs and Symptoms: Manganese deficiency has been associated with fragile bones, skin disorders, nausea, loss of weight, lowered fertility, and other problems. The deficiency is relatively rare, with the first case not being recognized until the early 1970s.

Where to Find It: Legumes, nuts, seeds, cereal grains, and leafy vegetables contain manganese. In general, foods of plant origin are better sources of this mineral than are foods that have come from animals.

Molybdenum

The very small amounts of molybdenum in the human body are found in the liver, bones, skin, kidney and other tissues. The body's supply of molybdenum rises or falls quickly with changes in diet that affect the intake of this mineral.

Molybdenum's Duties: Molybdenum aids in growth and development, and plays a role in a number of metabolic reactions.

Deficiency Signs and Symptoms: It cannot be said with certainty what a lack of molybdenum would do to humans, because deficiency symptoms have not been reported and studied. In animals, molybdenum deficiency causes anemia, weight loss, and stunted growth.

Where to Find It: Peas, beans, lentils, dark green, leafy vegetables, organ meats, and whole-grain breads contain molybdenum. The molybdenum content of fruits, vegetables, and grains varies according to the amount of molybdenum in the soil where they were grown.

Nickel

Although nickel is found in the blood, adrenal glands, bones, teeth, brain, lungs, kidney, and skin, its exact functions are not known. Still, the Food & Nutrition Board, which sets the RDAs, states that there is "substantial evidence to establish the essentiality" of nickel.

Nickel's Duties: Nickel is found within human RNA. (RNA is ribonucleic acid, a substance that helps to transmit genetic information within the body's cells.) The mineral is thought to activate a number of enzymes, and to help keep cell membranes and nucleic acids structurally sound.

Deficiency Signs and Symptoms: The signs and symptoms of a nickel deficiency in humans are not well known or understood.

Where to Find It and Other Vital Information: Vegetables and grains are better sources of nickel than are foods of animal origin.

Phosphorus

Widely available in foods, phosphorus is the second most abundant mineral in the body (calcium is the most abundant).

Like calcium, phosphorus accounts for a significant portion of body weight, with 1 to 1½ pounds of the average person's body weight being made up of phosphorus. Between 80 and 90 percent of the body's phosphorus is found in the bones and teeth, with the remainder playing important roles in every single cell in the body.

Phosphorus's Duties: Phosphorus has more known functions than any other mineral in the body. In addition to working with calcium to keep the bones and teeth strong, phosphorus helps to build cell walls and the soft tissues that make up the heart, brain, muscles, and kidneys. The mineral is also needed to convert fat, protein, and carbohydrates into energy, to ensure that the B-vitamins work, and to maintain the proper pH balance in the blood.

Deficiency Signs and Symptoms: Phosphorus deficiency, which is relatively rare, may cause anorexia, weakness, numbness, pains in the bones, fatigue, anxiety, and irritability.

Where to Find It and Other Information: Often associated with protein, phosphorus is found in meat, fish, poultry, and eggs, as well as in nuts, legumes, and grains. Milk is an excellent source of phosphorus because the mineral is best absorbed when calcium is present, and milk contains both. The average person takes in as much as 30 percent of his dietary phosphorus from food additives and soft drinks. Having too much phosphorus can upset the calcium-phosphorus balance and harm the bones.

Potassium

The average adult male body contains about 9 ounces of potassium, the average woman's body some 10 percent less. Much of it is found inside the body's cells, with smaller concentrations of the mineral in the fluid outside the cells.

Potassium's Duties: Together with chloride and sodium, potassium makes sure that the body fluids are properly balanced and distributed throughout the body. Potassium also helps to ensure that the muscles contract and relax properly, and that nerve impulses travel through the nervous system.

In addition, potassium plays a role in regulating blood pressure and the heart rhythm. And since potassium balances out some of the negative effects of excessive sodium, potassium-rich foods can be very beneficial for those who are eating the typical high-sodium diet. Potassium may also help to prevent strokes and certain forms of depression, as well as acne, swelling, fatigue, and nervousness.

Deficiency Signs and Symptoms: Potassium deficiency has been linked to low blood pressure, irregular heartbeat, elevated cholesterol, slow growth, fragile bones, kidney damage, breathing difficulties, acne, constipation, edema (excess fluid in the body), fatigue, weakness, depression, insomnia, and other difficulties.

Potassium deficiency, which is more often found among the elderly and hospitalized patients, may develop as the result of chronic vomiting or diarrhea, kidney disease, or excessive use of diuretics ("water pills") or laxatives.

Where to Find It: Potassium is found in whole grains, legumes, fruits, vegetables, and meat.

Selected Sources of Potassium

Food	Serving Size	Potassium (mg)
Figs, dried	10	1,332
Avocado, California	1 medium	1,208
Papaya	1 medium	780
Dates	10	541
Bulgur	1 c, parboiled	459
Banana	1 medium	550
Milk, skim	1 c	408
Cantaloupe	¼ melon	251
Guava	1	256
Orange juice, fresh	½ c	236
Apple	1 (with skin)	159
Apricot	1 raw	104
Provolone cheese	1 oz	39
Muenster cheese	1 oz	38

Selenium

Although discovered in the early 1800s, selenium was not recognized as an essential mineral for humans until the 1960s.

More years passed before medical researchers began to appreciate the mineral's potential for helping the body to resist cancer, heart disease, and the effects of aging.

Selenium's Duties: Serving as part of an enzyme called glutathione peroxidase, selenium is a powerful antioxidant that protects cell walls and red blood cells from oxidative damage. In addition, selenium strengthens the immune system, and helps to control the damaging effects of mercury and other toxic minerals that find their way into the body.

Deficiency Signs and Symptoms: Lack of selenium may lead to liver damage, elevated cholesterol, poor growth, and sterility in males. Low levels of selenium in the blood have also been linked to a greater risk of heart disease, stroke, and angina (chest pain associated with heart disease). Studies have shown that people with low levels of selenium in the blood tend to have more cancers of the breast, colon, rectum, lung, and other parts of the body. Those who live in areas where the soil is rich in selenium, and are presumably eating the selenium-rich food that grows in that soil, tend to have less cancer.

Where to Find It: Whole grains, poultry, meat, and fish are good sources of selenium. The mineral is also found in lesser amounts in vegetables and fruits. As noted above, the selenium in foods can vary widely, depending upon the selenium content of the soil in which it was grown.

Silicon

Silicon, which is concentrated in the skin and connective tissue, is a relatively new addition to the list of essential trace minerals. Although the mineral's exact duties are not fully understood, it appears to play a role in the calcification of bones, as well as in the building and maintenance of connective tissue.

Silicon's Duties: Silicon assists in the development of bones and connective tissue.

Deficiency Signs and Symptoms: The results of a silicon deficiency are difficult to identify, for silicon is widely available in food. Lack of silicon may lead to poorly developed bones.

Where to Find It: Silicon is found in vegetables, cooked dried peas and beans, and whole-grain cereals and breads.

Sodium

The typical adult body contains some four ounces of sodium, about two-thirds of which is found in body fluids, nerve, and muscle tissue. The rest is held in the bones.

Sodium's Duties: Together with chloride and potassium, sodium makes sure that body fluids are properly distributed throughout the body, that the pH balance is maintained, and that the nerves and muscles work properly. Sodium also helps metabolic materials pass through cell walls into the cells themselves, where they can be utilized.

Deficiency Signs and Symptoms: A lack of sodium may lead to abdominal cramps, dizziness, headaches, low blood pressure, infections, memory difficulties, seizures, loss of weight, fatigue, dizziness, confusion, and other problems. Sodium deficiency may develop with severe vomiting, diarrhea, or fasting. However, the more common problem is too much sodium, which has been associated with elevated blood pressure.

Where to Find It: Sodium is found in common table salt. Salt added to foods during processing or cooking, and at the table, is a major source of dietary sodium. Sodium is also found in milk, eggs, and a variety of vegetables and fruits, such as carrots, cantaloupe, and dried apricots.

Sulfur

Sulfur is found throughout the body, especially in the skin, muscles, hair, joints, and nails. A component of four amino acids (cysteine, cystine, methionine, and taurine), sulfur is found wherever there are large concentrations of protein.

Sulfur's Duties: Sulfur helps proteins maintain their structure (and hair to curl). It plays a role in various enzyme systems, in the body's ability to utilize energy, in the elimination of certain toxic substances from the body, and in blood clotting. It is also a constituent of some B-vitamins, insulin, and collagen.

Deficiency Signs and Symptoms: Sulfur deficiencies are uncommon in this country, and their signs and symptoms not well recognized.

Where to Find It: Sulfur is found in meat, poultry, fish, eggs, milk, milk products, and other foods containing good amounts of protein.

Tin

Tin is considered by some experts to be an essential trace mineral. Highest concentrations are found in the teeth and bones, with the rest distributed to the lungs, liver, heart, muscles, and other body tissues.

Tin's Duties: Tin plays a role in helping proteins and other large molecules to maintain their structures. The mineral also functions in enzyme systems that help to regulate cellular metabolism.

Deficiency Signs and Symptoms: Animals fed diets low in tin have suffered from slow growth and reproductive difficulties.

Where to Find It: Good sources of dietary tin include organ meats and whole grains. A fair portion of the tin we consume is leached from the surface of unlacquered tin cans containing orange juice, tomato sauce, pineapple or pineapple juice, and the like.

Zinc

Although zinc has been known to be essential to microorganisms for a century, and essential to rats for half a century, it has only recently been declared essential to humans.

Zinc's Duties: Zinc plays many roles in the body. In addition to strengthening the immune system and memory, and aiding in sex and reproduction, zinc helps to keep the bones strong and blood cholesterol at normal levels. Zinc keeps the blood sugar in check by helping to ensure that insulin performs properly. It also plays a role in body growth and development, plus the maintenance of proper blood pressure and heart rhythms. Acting as an antioxidant, zinc protects the macula, which is in the center of the retina, from oxidative damage that can destroy vision.

Deficiency Signs and Symptoms: Zinc deficiency may cause acne, anorexia, slow growth, delayed sexual maturity, diarrhea, eczema, fatigue, elevated cholesterol, impotence and male infertility, increased infections, deterioration of the vision, apathy, depression, irritability, memory impairment, paranoia, amnesia, and poor healing of wounds. Zinc intake is commonly inadequate in the American diet.

Where to Find It: Zinc is found in oysters and other seafood, meat and eggs, and in lesser amounts in whole grains, peas, beans, and lentils.

Selected Sources of Zinc

Food	Serving Size	Zinc (mg)
Oysters	3 oz, raw	63.0
Calf's liver	3 oz, cooked	7.0
Wheat germ	1 oz	5.0
Pumpkin seeds	1 oz	3.0
Sardines	3 oz, canned	2.0
Yogurt, plain	1 c	1.3
Egg	1 large	0.7

OTHER MINERALS

Other minerals, including boron, vanadium, and cadmium are also found in the body. The Food & Nutrition Board, which sets the RDAs, feels that there is *substantial evidence* backing the idea that some currently ''nonessential'' minerals are vital, so they may someday be moved to the list of essential minerals.

Recent evidence indicates that boron plays an important role in human health. Boron helps to keep the bones healthy by preventing excessive amounts of calcium from escaping the body. Even if the diet is high in calcium, without boron to ''hold the calcium in,'' it may leave the body and the bones may weaken. Boron also plays an important role in mental alertness. People eating boron-deficient diets tend to perform poorly on simple tasks, but the problems disappear when they are given boron supplements. Boron may also reduce the symptoms of menopause. Apples, peaches, grapes, legumes, pears, honey, peanuts, hazelnuts, and almonds all contain good amounts of boron.

Although other minerals, such as arsenic and lead, have long been thought to be poisonous, small amounts may prove to be necessary for human life or health. For example, animals fed diets deficient in arsenic, lead, or lithium suffer from slow growth and difficulty reproducing. More research will undoubtedly clarify their roles in human health and life.

THE MINERAL TEAM

Although the minerals have been individually analyzed and discussed, they work together as a team to build good health. There may be much more calcium than zinc in the body, for example, but each has an important role to play. The larger effect of the minerals working together, and working with the other nutrients, is much greater than the sum of the individual parts. For example:

- Phosphorus and molybdenum work with the B-vitamins to extract energy from food.
- Sulfur is part of vitamin B_1.
- Cobalt is found in B_{12}.
- Chromium and niacin work together to make the glucose tolerance factor (GTF).
- Copper helps the body absorb and utilize iron.
- Selenium and vitamin E work closely together, as antioxidants, to protect the heart and guard against cancer.

Too much of a good thing, however, can be dangerous, so the minerals must be kept in balance. For example:

- Excess calcium can upset the calcium-magnesium balance and encourage heart disease.
- Iron, zinc, and calcium compete to be absorbed in the intestine. Only so much can "get through," so excessive intake of one could lead to a deficiency of another.

Balance is the key to good nutrient teamwork, which is why it's important not to overlook or to overemphasize the importants of nutrients. Taking massive doses of calcium to keep the bones strong, for example, won't help much if you don't have enough vitamin D and phosphorus to ensure the proper absorption and utilization of calcium. And to make matters worse, large amounts of calcium can upset the calcium-magnesium balance, which helps to regulate the cardiovascular system.

How can you ensure that your mineral team is balanced? No single food contains all the nutrients and phytochemicals needed for vibrant health, so the best approach is to eat a wide variety of foods, with special emphasis on fresh vegetables and fruits, plus whole grains. (See the guidelines on page 42.)

THE RECOMMENDED DAILY ALLOWANCES FOR MINERALS

To help people determine how much of each essential nutrient is needed for good health and growth, the Food & Nutrition Board has established Recommended Daily Allowances (RDAs) for several essential nutrients. See figure 3.1 on pages 68 and 69 for the RDAs for minerals.

In addition, the Food & Nutrition Board has devised a table of "safe and adequate daily dietary intakes" for copper, manganese, fluoride, chromium, and molybdenum. The intake ranges are:

Figure 3.2. Estimated Safe and Adequate
Daily Dietary Intakes of Selected Minerals

Category	Age (years)	Copper (mg)	Manganese (mg)	Fluoride (mg)	Chromium (mcg)	Molybdenum (mcg)
Infants	0–0.5	0.4–0.6	0.6–0.6	0.1–0.5	10–40	15–30
	0.5–1	0.6–0.7	0.6–1.0	0.2–1.0	20–60	20–40
Children and adolescents	1–3	0.7–1.0	1.0–1.5	0.5–1.5	20–80	25–50
	4–6	1.0–1.5	1.5–2.0	1.0–2.5	30–120	30–75
	7–10	1.0–2.0	2.0–3.0	1.5–2.5	50–200	50–150
	11+	1.5–2.5	2.0–5.0	1.5–2.5	50–200	75–250
Adults	18+	1.5–3.0	2.0–5.0	1.5–4.0	50–200	75–250

The RDAs and the "safe and adequate daily dietary intakes" are only guidelines, or estimates of a healthy person's needs. The RDAs are set too low. While sufficient to stave off disease, they do not promote optimal health.

Caution: Too much of a mineral can, in some cases, be as damaging as not enough. Here are some of the signs and symptoms of mineral toxicity:

Calcium: Excess calcium may lead to anorexia, depression, memory impairment, muscle weakness, and other problems. Too much calcium can also interfere with the absorption of iron and zinc.

Chromium: An "overdose" of chromium may lead to skin problems, ulcers, liver and kidney damage.

Cobalt: Ingesting excess amounts of inorganic cobalt, which is not bound up in vitamin B_{12}, may lead to heart disorders and an overproduction of red blood cells. Drinking large amounts of beer may induce these rare symptoms, for cobalt is used in the manufacture of some beers.

Copper: Copper's toxic symptoms include muscle and joint pain, depression, nervousness and irritability.

Fluoride: Taking in too much fluoride may lead to pitting and mottling of the teeth. Large intakes can produce symptoms similar to those of arthritis, and very extreme cases of fluoride excess can cause death.

Iodine: Iodine "overdose" can produce the same thing that adequate amounts prevent: goiter.

Iron: The body does not excrete excess iron. Instead, it simply stops absorbing iron from food when it has enough. However, it is possible for iron stores in the body to build to excess, especially in men. This may lead to many problems, such as headaches, fatigue, dizziness, and anorexia, and even heart disease.

Magnesium: Magnesium "overload" is unlikely, for the kidneys are very good at excreting excesses of this mineral. Toxic symptoms of magnesium excess include irregular heart rhythms, low blood pressure, muscle weakness, fatigue, thirst, and other difficulties.

Manganese: Too much manganese may lead to hallucinations, insomnia, muscle pains, nerve disorders, and anorexia. It may also interfere with the absorption of iron, leading to an iron-deficiency anemia.

Molybdenum: Excess consumption may lead to pain and swelling of the joints.

Phosphorus: Those who consume large amounts of soft

Figure 3.1. RDA for Minerals

Food & Nutrition Board, National Academy of Sciences—National Research Council
Recommended Dietary Allowances. Revised 1989.

Minerals

	Age	Calcium (mg)	Phosphorus (mg)	Magnesium (mg)	Iron (mg)	Zinc (mg)	Iodine (mcg)	Selenium (mcg)
Infants	0.0–0.5	400	300	40	6	5	40	10
	0.5–1.0	600	500	60	10	5	50	15
Children	1–3	800	800	80	10	10	70	20
	4–6	800	800	120	10	10	90	20
	7–10	800	800	170	10	10	120	30
Males	11–14	1,200	1,200	270	12	15	150	40
	15–18	1,200	1,200	400	12	15	150	50
	19–24	1,200	1,200	350	10	15	150	70
	25–50	800	800	350	10	15	150	70
	51+	800	800	350	10	15	150	70

Females							
11–14	1,200	1,200	280	15	12	150	45
15–18	1,200	1,200	300	15	12	150	50
19–24	1,200	1,200	280	15	12	150	55
25–50	800	800	280	15	12	150	55
51+	800	800	280	10	12	150	55
Pregnant	1,200	1,200	300	30	15	175	65
Lactating[1]	1,200	1,200	355	15	19	200	75

[1]Although the RDAs are given separately for the first and second six months of lactation, I've included only the figures for the first six months, which are slightly higher in a few categories.

drinks, convenience foods and meat, but relatively few cal-
cium-containing foods, can develop an imbalance in the cal-
cium-to-phosphorus ratio. This may lead to osteoporosis.

Potassium: Excess potassium in the body may produce
weakness, kidney failure, muscle breakdown, memory difficulties, and other problems.

Selenium: A great many ailments have been associated with
selenium excess, including arthritis, diabetes, fatigue, suppres-
sion of the immune system, impairment of the liver and kidneys, nausea, and skin problems.

Sodium: The most famous result of sodium "overdose" is
high blood pressure. Other potential problems include congestive heart failure, swelling, seizures, tremors, and hyperactiv-
ity.

Zinc: Taking in too much zinc can interfere with the body's
ability to absorb copper from food. Large intakes can harm
the immune system, and increase the risk of heart disease by
lowering the HDL ("good") cholesterol. Other symptoms of
excess include nausea and vomiting.

Caution: *Taking mineral supplements might be dangerous
if you are also taking medications. For example, taking a
calcium supplement while you are using iron preparations
such as Feosol™ or Mol-Iron™ for anemia may reduce the
amount of iron absorbed. And iron supplements may reduce
the effectiveness of thyroid replacement hormones such as
Synthroid.™ These are just some of the potential supplement medication interactions. Be sure to tell your physician
if you are taking any vitamins or other supplements.*

CHAPTER 4

The Healing Powers of
Phytochemicals

Some of the most exciting nutritional research being conducted in research centers around the world has to do with a large number of previously overlooked substances in foods. Neither vitamins nor minerals, they are called phytochemicals (*phyto* means "from plants"). There are hundreds of phytochemicals, from the familiar chlorophyll that gives green vegetables their color to the exotic genistein, a factor found in soy foods that can "starve" cancer cells by interfering with their blood supply.

We used to think that only the vitamins, minerals, protein, fat, carbohydrates, and fiber in foods were important. Now we know that hundreds of other minute substances help to strengthen the immune system, fight off cancer, keep the coronary arteries clear, beat back infections, prevent oxidation, delay the symptoms of aging, and otherwise help to keep us healthy. Let's take a brief look at a few of the many phytochemicals that are revolutionizing the field of nutrition.

MIRACULOUS "MEDICINES" IN FOODS

Adenosine: A natural substance found in onions, garlic, and black mushrooms, adenosine can help protect against heart disease and stroke by "thinning" the blood. "Thin" blood is less likely to produce clots that can lodge in an artery supplying blood to the heart or brain, triggering a heart attack or stroke.

Ajoene: A powerful blood thinner found in garlic that, like adenosine, can help to prevent strokes and heart disease.

Allicin: The strong-smelling substance in garlic, allicin is a natural antibiotic.

Alpha-linolenic Acid: This is an omega-3 fatty acid found in olive oil, canola oil, and flaxseed oil that is believed to protect against heart disease. People eating a Mediterranean diet tend to have much less heart disease than do those eating the standard American fare. That may be because the typical Mediterranean diet has more alpha-linolenic acid than the American diet. Alpha-linolenic acid may also guard against cancer and arthritis.

Antioxidants: Although the oxygen we constantly breathe in gives us life, it is also a highly reactive substance that can be quite damaging to the body if allowed to "run wild." (See the discussion of oxidation and free radicals on page 2.)

The body's natural defenses against oxidation are aided by antioxidants from food, including beta-carotene, vitamins C and E, the mineral selenium, and phytochemicals such as glutathione, lycopene, and quercetin. Many researchers now believe that controlling the oxidants is the key to preventing a great deal of heart disease, cancer, arthritis, and other diseases, and many of the ravages of aging.

Bioflavonoids: See "Other Vitamin-like Substances" in Chapter 2.

Capsaicin: The "hot" part of hot chili peppers, capsaicin helps to relieve respiratory ailments by clearing away mucus clogging up the breathing tubes. It also protects against stomach ulcers, and is used as an ointment to lessen the pain of arthritis and shingles. (Capsaicin apparently blocks pain by temporarily "burning out" nerve cells, preventing pain messages from getting through.) The "hot stuff" also has anti-inflammatory properties.

Carnitine: Made from amino acids in the liver, kidney, and brain, carnitine is a vitamin-like compound that plays an important role in the conversion of fat into energy in the body cells. Carnitine increases good cholesterol, while lowering the bad. A deficiency has been linked to various heart disorders, which can be treated with carnitine supplementation.

Catechins: These bioflavonoids help the body to fight off cancer, and possibly viruses as well. (See the "Bioflavonoids" entry under "Other Vitamin-like Substances" in Chapter 2.)

Chlorophyll: In addition to giving green vegetables their color, chlorophyll is a proven antimutagen that guards against the alteration of cellular DNA. Chlorophyll is believed by some researchers to block initiation, the first step in the transformation of normal cells to cancerous killers. The green-colored phytochemical is also an antioxidant.

Coenzyme Q₁₀: See the "Ubiquinone" entry under "Other Vitamin-like Substances" in Chapter 2.

Coumarins: Natural blood thinners, the coumarins guard against heart attacks by preventing the formation of unnecessary blood clots that can dam up the coronary arteries. Keeping the blood thin also reduces the risk of strokes and other problems related to blood that clots too easily. Coumarins are found in fresh vegetables, fruits, and cereal grains.

Ellagic Acid: Found in strawberries, grapes and cherries, ellagic acid disarms carcinogens before they can make healthy cells cancerous.

Free Radicals: See the "Antioxidants" entry.

Genistein: Cancer cells need a steady supply of fresh blood in order to survive and thrive. Genistein checks the growth of some cancers by interfering with the blood supply to tumors. It is found in soy and soy-based products.

Glutathione: A naturally occurring antioxidant, glutathione is believed to protect the body against many carcinogens and may help to slow the aging process. Glutathione is found in avocados, watermelon, strawberries, tomatoes, and other common foods.

Hesperidin: See the "Bioflavonoids" entry under "Other Vitamin-like Substances" in Chapter 2.

Indoles: Found in cabbage, broccoli, Brussels sprouts, cauliflower and other members of the cruciferous family of vegetables, indoles are powerful anticancer compounds that help to protect against breast, colon, and other cancers.

Isoflavones: Certain types of tumors need estrogen in order to grow. But the estrogen can't "help" the tumors unless it can "park" in specific estrogen receptors on tumor cells. Isoflavones can prevent the tumors from growing by shoving themselves into the estrogen "parking spaces," leaving no place for the estrogen. Isoflavones are found in peas, beans, and lentils.

Lignans: As both antioxidants and deactivators of estrogen, lignans help to protect body cells and to slow down the growth of certain tumors.

Limonene: As the name suggests, limonene is found in limes and other citrus fruits. Limonene helps to prevent or slow the growth of certain cancers.

Lipoic Acid: See the "Other Vitamin-like Substances" section in Chapter 2.

Lutein: A cousin to beta-carotene, lutein is a carotenoid and an antioxidant found in dark green, leafy vegetables such as kale and spinach.

Lycopene: A naturally occurring antioxidant found in tomatoes, watermelon, and other foods, lycopene is a carotenoid. Research on the diets of cancer patients suggests that this relatively unknown carotenoid may help the body ward off colon and bladder cancer.

Monoterpenes: These are naturally occurring antioxidants found in broccoli, cabbage, carrots, and other vegetables and fruits.

Phenols: Also known as phenolic acids, the phenols are a remarkable group of substances found in fruits, potatoes, some nuts, garlic, and green tea. The phenols have antiviral properties. As powerful antioxidants, they protect against heart disease, cancer, and other ailments. At least one of the phenols, ellagic acid, helps to control excessive bleeding in humans, and has been shown to reduce blood pressure in animal studies.

The phenols also guard against cancer by neutralizing certain carcinogens, suppressing the promotion of activated cells, and increasing the production of natural detoxifying substances (such as the powerful detoxifer glutathione).

There are over 200 phenols, with names such as caffeic acid, chlorogenic acid, cinamic acid, ellagic acid, ferulic acid, and gallotannic acid.

Phytates: Phytates are compounds that help to prevent the growth of steroid-dependent tumors. Found in cereal grains and other foods, the phytates can be harmful if taken in excess, for they can reduce the body's ability to absorb calcium and other minerals from food.

Phytoestrogens: Sometimes called "almost estrogens," phytoestrogens are substances found in plants that have weak estrogen-like activity. They bind to estrogen receptors in certain cells, locking the estrogen out and preventing the hormone from interacting with the cells.

Breast cancer requires estrogen to flourish. But when phytoestrogens bind to the cancer cells, they lock out the real estrogen cancer needs. Studies have shown that people who eat large amounts of phytoestrogen-containing foods, such as soy products and beans, are less likely to develop breast cancer, or to succumb to cancer of the pancreas.

Protease Inhibitors: Found in beans, whole grains, and other foods, the protease inhibitors help normal cells to resist the DNA damage that can turn them cancerous.

Quercetin: A bioflavonoid and naturally occurring antioxidant found in red grapes, red and yellow onions, broccoli, and other foods.

Resveratrol: A substance found in the skins of red and white grapes that helps to prevent the unnecessary blood clots that can trigger serious problems such as a heart attack or stroke. Resveratrol is found in red wine and red grape juice. (It is not found in white wine, because the grape skins, which contain the resveratrol, are discarded early in the manufacturing process.)

Rutin: See the "Bioflavonoids" entry under "Other Vitamin-like Substances" in Chapter 2.

Sulfides: Like the phytates, sulfides protect against steroid-dependent tumors. Found in garlic, as well as in cabbage, broccoli, Brussels sprouts and other members of the crucifer family, sulfides may also protect against heart disease and strokes by thinning the blood and reducing blood pressure.

Tannins: One of the substances in tea that helps to keep arteries healthy by keeping the blood "thin." They also have anti-inflamatory properties.

Taurine: An amino acid that protects against irregular heartbeat, taurine has antioxidant properties, and may help to control blood pressure.

Terpenes: Found in lemons and other foods, the terpenes help to keep cholesterol under control and prevent or slow the growth of certain cancers.

Ubiquinone: Also known as Coenzyme Q_{10}. See the "Other Vitamin-like Substances" section in Chapter 2.

Zeaxantin: A carotenoid found in spinach and other dark green, leafy vegetables, it may play a leading role in protecting the eyes from the progressive loss of vision caused by age-related macular degeneration.

Abbreviation and Conversion Table

oz	=	ounce
c	=	cup
gm	=	gram
mg	=	milligram
mcg	=	microgram
IU	=	International Units

Conversion/Equivalents for
Grams, Milligrams, and Micrograms

1 gm = 1,000 mg
1 mg = 1,000 mcg

CHAPTER 5

Natural Healing with Foods,
A to Z

*Let food be your medicine, and medicine be your
food.*

—HIPPOCRATES

Knowing about the vitamins, minerals, and phytochemicals
found in foods is a wonderful start. In this chapter we'll take
the next step, looking at nearly 100 foods: where they're from,
what's in them, and how they can help to keep us healthy.

In days of old, physicians said: "Show me what a man eats,
and I'll tell you his disease." We've learned a lot more about
foods since then. Perhaps in the near future we'll be able to
say: "Show me what people eat, and I'll tell you how healthy
they are."

We're not yet able to promise that eating certain foods will
guarantee optimal health, but a tremendous amount of scientific research has shown that healthful eating strengthens the
immune system, lowers the risk of killer diseases such as cancer and heart disease, and helps to keep us energetic and
healthy throughout a long life.

READING THE FOOD PROFILE BOXES

The "Food Profile" boxes following the discussion of each
food in this chapter present the RDAs (Recommended Dietary

Allowances) for the vitamins and minerals in that food. The percentages given are based on the 1989 RDAs published by the National Research Council's Food & Nutrition Board. These percentages may be different from figures you have seen in other books because there is more than one RDA for each vitamin and mineral. Indeed, the RDAs are given in 18 different categories, depending on age, sex, and whether one is pregnant or lactating. And some nutrients do not have RDAs. Instead, they have "Estimated Safe and Adequate Daily Dietary Intakes" given in either numbers or ranges for seven different age groups.

To simplify matters, I chose a single figure for each vitamin and mineral. After setting aside the figures for pregnant and lactating women, I selected the highest remaining figure for each nutrient as the basis for my calculations. And when computing the RDAs, I rounded up.

The mineral potassium has neither an RDA nor an "Estimated Safe and Adequate Daily Dietary Intake." That's why "NA," meaning non-applicable, follows potassium in the food profiles.

A quick note on beta carotene, the "plant form" of vitamin A. Although fruits, vegetables, and grains contain beta carotene rather than vitamin A, I've followed standard conventions and listed the nutrient as "Vitamin A" in the nutrient breakdowns that follow each food in Chapter 5.

Finally, I used the Food & Nutrition Board's recommendations as the basis for my suggestions for how many servings of fruits, vegetables, and other foods one should have per day. The Food & Nutrition Board's guidelines are both sensible and attainable, neither too "strict" nor too lax. They include:

- Eat a variety of foods
- Eat 5 or more servings a day of vegetables and fruits, especially citrus fruits, and green and yellow vegetables
- Eat 6 or more servings a day of peas, beans, breads, and other foods high in complex carbohydrates

In the following profiles, the adjectives I use to describe the nutrients content of foods have specific meanings:

A *"good"* source means the food contains 10 to 24 percent of the RDA;

A *"very good"* source means the food contains 25 to 49 percent of the RDA;

An *"excellent"* source means the food contains 50–99 percent of the RDA;

A *"tremendous"* source means the food contains more than 100 percent of the RDA.

Keep these abbreviations in mind as you read through the food profiles:

- gm = gram
- mg = milligram
- mcg = microgram
- IU = International Unit
- RE = Retinol equivalent, a measure of vitamin A activity
- NA = not applicable. This is only used after potassium, because there is neither an RDA nor an "Estimated Safe and Adequate Daily Dietary Allowance" for this mineral.

 ## ALFALFA SPROUTS

Although many people think that alfalfa is related to grass, it's actually a member of the pea family. Most of the alfalfa grown in this country is used as livestock feed, but the long, thin, green-tipped alfalfa sprouts have been served in salads and sandwiches at "health food" restaurants for many years. Alfalfa sprouts have been used as an herbal healer for numerous ailments, including constipation, skin disorders, and "tired blood."

Alfalfa's Healing Properties

Low in fat and calories, high in fiber, alfalfa sprouts help:

• Lower cholesterol

In addition, the sprouts contain carotenes and chlorophyll. Carotenes are a group of some 400 naturally occurring food pigments, many of which strengthen the immune system, fight off tumors, and control the dangerous oxidation reactions that can harm the body. (Beta-carotene is the best known of the carotenes.) Chlorophyll, the green pigment found in foods, also has antioxidant and anticancer properties.

What Scientists Have Learned About Alfalfa Sprouts

Alfalfa Sprouts & Cholesterol: Alfalfa has shown itself to be an effective anticholesterol agent. In a study of people with elevated cholesterol, giving 1.4 oz of sprouted alfalfa seeds three times a day for eight weeks caused the total cholesterol to fall by over 15 percent. The bad LDL cholesterol also dropped significantly.

Alfalfa, Vitamin K, and the Blood: Alfalfa sprouts contain the relatively "unknown" vitamin K, whose primary duty is to regulate the body's blood clotting mechanisms. A lack of K can lead to slow clotting time, which means one may bleed excessively when injured. Vitamin K also helps the body to retain its calcium, thus keeping the bones strong. In addition, researchers feel that vitamin K might help to slow the growth of cancers of the stomach, bladder, liver, kidney, breast, ovary, and colon.

Including the Food in Your Diet

Regularly top off your salads with alfalfa sprouts, and add them to your sandwiches. It's a quick and tasty way to help keep your cholesterol low and your vitamin K stores high.

> **Caution:** *Eating alfalfa sprouts can cause a lupus-like syndrome in certain people. Those with autoimmune diseases such as lupus or rheumatoid arthritis should carefully discuss with their physicians whether they should eat alfalfa sprouts.*

```
ALFALFA SPROUTS
1 cup

Calories          10
Protein           1.3 gm
Carbohydrate      1.3 gm
Fat               0.2 gm
Cholesterol       0   mg
Dietary Fiber     0.7 gm

                  Amount              RDA
Folacin           11.9 mcg            6%
```

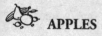 **APPLES**

*Eat an apple on going to bed, and you'll keep
the doctor from earning his bread.*
—ENGLISH PROVERB

The history of apples is perhaps as long as the history of mankind. Fossilized remains of apples have been found in the ruins of ancient settlements dating back some five thousand years.

Often called "the king of fruits," apples have played an important role in American folklore. Johnny Appleseed spent forty years planting apple orchards all around the Ohio River area during the early part of the nineteenth century. The lyrics of a twentieth-century Broadway musical urged us to "eat an apple every day," and every school child knows that "an apple a day keeps the doctor away."

Apples have also played a distinguished role in health and healing. Documents found in ancient Egyptian pyramids and tombs praise the apple's medicinal qualities. Through the years, apples have been prescribed for nervous conditions, skin problems, gout, liver troubles, and gallbladder disease.

Although there are over 7,000 varieties of apple, a mere eight (Golden Delicious, Red Delicious, Granny Smith, Jonathan, McIntosh, Rome Beauty, Stayman, and York) account for 80 percent of all the apples grown in the United States.

The Apple's Healing Properties

Although apples are not as high in vitamins or minerals as many other fruits, they contain a variety of nutrients and phytochemicals, including soluble fiber, boron, iron, vitamin B_2, and potassium. It is fortunate that Americans enjoy them (eating some 40 pounds per person every year) because apples:

- Fight cancer
- Protect the heart and cardiovascular system
- Lower cholesterol
- Keep blood sugar under control
- Have antibacterial and antiviral properties
- May help to keep bones strong
- Help to relieve menopausal symptoms in some women

In addition, apples can assist in weight control by suppressing the appetite, and they help to relieve constipation.

What Scientists Have Learned About the Apple

Apples and Cancer: Epidemiologists (scientists who study large groups of people) have long known that those who eat diets high in fruits and vegetables tend to have less cancer overall. Study has shown that even amongst the Cajuns in Louisiana, whose diets include tremendous amounts of pork, bacon, sausage, ham, and other foods associated with pancreatic and other cancers, fruit has a protective effect. Cajuns who ate the most fruit had the least pancreatic cancer, even *if they did not cut back on their intake of cured meats.*

How do apples and other fruits fight cancer? Part of fruit's anticancer effects stem from the various phenols that they contain. Phenols neutralize certain carcinogens, inhibit the transformation of precancerous cells into cancerous bodies, and spur the body's natural production of anticancer substances. (One of these cancer-fighters is glutathione, which detoxifies cancer-causing substances inside the body.) Apples have good amounts of the anticancer phenol called *chlorogenic acid,* as well as a biologically active phenol named *cinamic acid.*

Apples have a second way of fighting cancer. They contain a soluble fiber called pectin, which reduces the risk of colon cancer. In studies conducted at the University of Texas Health Sciences Center, feeding laboratory animals pectin lowered the rate of colon cancer by up to 50 percent.

There may be another way in which apples help to defeat colon cancer. Aspirin (salicylic acid) has recently been shown to be a colon-cancer fighter. Apples are among the foods with the greatest amounts of salicylates, the natural substance from which aspirin is derived. More research is needed before we can say that the apple's aspirin-like effects prevent colon cancer, but this is certainly a promising avenue of inquiry.

Apples and Heart Disease: The pectin and other soluble fibers in apples play a large role in reducing total cholesterol and the LDL ("bad") cholesterol, although exactly how they do this is not yet fully understood. In one study, 30 healthy volunteers were asked to eat two to three apples a day. At the end of the month-long trial, total cholesterol levels had dropped significantly in 80 percent of the subjects. In addition, the bad cholesterol dropped and the good cholesterol rose. This finding has been duplicated in many other studies conducted in laboratories around the world.

Some of these pectin-cholesterol studies used whole apples, while others utilized pectin capsules. It appears that the whole apple does a better job of improving cholesterol profiles than do pectin capsules alone. This suggests that there is something else in the apple, besides the pectin, that keeps the bad cholesterol down and the good cholesterol up.

Apples, Diabetes and Blood Sugar: Diabetes mellitus is a serious, chronic disorder of metabolism afflicting some 14 million Americans. With diabetes, either the body does not make enough of the hormone called insulin, or body cells are unable to respond to insulin's order to accept sugar (glucose) from the bloodstream. In either case, body cells run short of sugar to burn for energy. Desperate, the diabetic body begins to burn up fat and protein for fuel. But it cannot completely burn the fat, leaving behind what are known as *ketone bodies.* Leftover ketone bodies accumulate, making the blood more acidic. This overly acidic blood (a condition called *keto-acidosis*) can lead to coma and death.

Before that happens, however, the changes in body chemistry brought about by diabetes damage small blood vessels and nerves throughout the body. Depending upon which vessels and nerves are damaged, the results can be skin problems, numbness of the hands and feet, blindness, kidney failure, stroke, impotence in men, sterility in women, and, in both sexes, an increased risk of heart attacks.

Fortunately, the pectin and other substances in apples help to reduce the harmful side effects of diabetes by keeping the blood sugar under control. One study, looking at the effect of pectin on blood sugar, found that giving insulin-dependent diabetics a ''milk shake'' containing the amount of pectin found in two apples, significantly reduced their need for the insulin they normally had to take after eating.

This and similar studies show that despite the natural sugar in apples, the fruit assists in the battle against diabetes by helping to keep blood sugar under control.

Apples and Infections: Over 30 years ago, researchers studied the health and dietary records of 1,300 students at Michigan State University. They found that the young men and women who ate the most apples had fewer infections of the upper respiratory tract, suffered from less tension, and were healthier in general than their peers who ate fewer apples. This observation was given scientific backing in the 1970s, when Canadian researchers found that extracts of apple and other fruits destroyed viruses in laboratory experiments. Although apples are not a specific cure for specific viruses, phenols and other substances in apples help to strengthen the immune system and increase one's resistance to viruses, bacteria, and other ''germs.''

Apples, Boron, Arthritis, and Menopause: Arthritis, the name given to any joint inflammation, is characterized by joint swelling and pain. The most common form of arthritis is osteoarthritis, which accounts for approximately 80 percent of all arthritis cases, and affects more than 15 million Americans. Osteoarthritis is caused by a breakdown of the smooth cartilage that cushions the ends of the bones where they meet to form a joint. As the cartilage deteriorates, the bones rub painfully together. (Almost everyone over the age of 60 has at least some signs of the disease.)

The mineral boron plays a vital role in bone health. In a study examining the mineral's impact on arthritis, 15 patients suffering from osteoarthritis were given either 6 mg of boron a day, or a placebo. Eight weeks later, the patients receiving boron reported a significant reduction in pain, and a feeling of improvement in their joints. Many studies of large populations in various countries have found that the more boron there is in the soil, the less osteoarthritis the people have. This is because foods grown in boron-rich soil tend to have more boron than do foods grown elsewhere. We may not know the boron content of the soil in which our food is grown, but we can eat as many boron-rich foods as possible, including apples, pears, grapes, peaches, almonds, peanuts, and honey.

Studies conducted by the U.S. Department of Agriculture have shown that eating plenty of foods containing boron can increase estrogen levels in postmenopausal women. Although more studies are required before definitive claims can be made, some researchers feel that eating a diet rich in boron-containing foods such as apples may eliminate the need for estrogen supplements in many women.

Including the Food in Your Diet

The Food & Nutrition Board recommends eating five or more servings of fruits and vegetables per day. An apple a day will help to fulfill this requirement, increase your resistance to a variety of diseases, and help keep the doctor away.

A lot of the pectin in apples is found in the peel, so think twice before removing and discarding it.

APPLE
1, with skin (approx. 5 oz)

Calories	81
Protein	0.3 gm
Carbohydrate	21.1 gm
Fat	0.5 gm
Cholesterol	0 mg
Dietary Fat	2.8 gm

	Amount	RDA
Vitamin C	7.9 mg	13%
Vitamin E	0.8 mg	8%

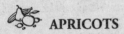 APRICOTS

Born in China some four thousand years ago, the apricot was widely distributed throughout Asia in ancient times. Alexander the Great is said to have brought the apricot to Greece, and from there it spread through Europe. The little peach-cousin arrived in California with the Spanish in the eighteenth century, and Americans quickly took to the delicious fruit. NASA even sent the apricot to the moon, as part of the astronaut's diet.

The Apricot's Healing Properties

Although small, apricots are good sources of beta-carotene and vitamin C. They also contain smaller amounts of potassium, iron, and fiber.

Apricot pits are the source of laetrile, a controversial drug that some have claimed cures cancer. Although there is a great deal of doubt over the effectiveness of laetrile, the beta-carotene and vitamin C in apricots *are* genuine cancer fighters. Both beta-carotene and vitamin C are antioxidants, which strengthen the body's resistance to cancer by controlling the oxidative damage that can turn normal cells cancerous. Both of these substances also strengthen the immune system, which is the body's primary defense against all types of cancer.

The fiber contained in apricots aids in the prevention of colon cancer. By making the stool bulkier and by moving it more rapidly through the intestines, fiber helps to dilute carcinogens in the stool, while reducing their exposure to cells lining the colon. In addition, dietary fiber reduces or eliminates constipation, hemorrhoids, varicose veins, and diverticular disease that often result from straining to eliminate.

Apricots also contain salicylate, the natural ingredient from which aspirin was originally derived. Future studies may find that apricots have analgesic and anti-inflammatory properties.

Including the Food in Your Diet

Health experts recommend eating five or more servings of fruit and vegetables a day. Regularly making an apricot part of your daily fruit intake will help to boost your immune system and your resistance to a variety of diseases.

People with a tendency toward calcium-oxalate stones may need to avoid or restrict their intake of apricots, and should discuss this with their physicians. Eating large amounts of apricots may cause some to suffer from gas.

	APRICOTS **3 (approx. 4 oz)**	
Calories	51	
Protein	1.5 gm	
Carbohydrate	11.8 gm	
Fat	0.5 gm	
Saturated Fat	———	
Dietary Fiber	1.4 gm	
	Amount	RDA
Vitamin A	227 RE	23%
Vitamin C	10.6 gm	17%
Iron	.6 mg	4%
Potassium	3.3 mg	NA

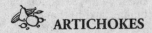 **ARTICHOKES**

The artichoke has long been popular throughout Europe. In fact, Pliny, the ancient Roman writer, noted that artichokes were highly esteemed and very expensive in the marketplace.

Although there are over 40 varieties of artichokes, the Italian green globe variety is far and away the most popular. The Jerusalem artichoke, however, is not an artichoke at all. Rather, it is a relative of the sunflower, and resembles jicama.

The Artichoke's Healing Properties

Artichokes are a very good source of folate, and a good source of magnesium, iron, and vitamin C. Very low in calories, they may:

• Slightly reduce cholesterol levels

What Scientists Have Learned About Artichokes

Artichokes and Cholesterol: Although their health effects have not been widely studied in recent years, studies conducted in the 1940s revealed that artichokes reduced cholesterol. Later studies, both in this country and abroad, confirmed that eating artichokes could lower cholesterol levels a bit. Pharmaceutical researchers have since used a substance in artichokes called cynarin as the basis for a cholesterol-lowering drug.

Including the Food in Your Diet

Making artichokes a regular part of the five or more daily servings of vegetables and fruits recommended by the Food & Nutrition Board will help to keep your heart healthy and immune system strong.

Enjoy the natural taste of artichokes, or at least keep the seasoning to a minimum. Drenching artichokes in butter turns an otherwise low-fat, low-cholesterol meal into a heart-stressor.

ARTICHOKE
1 boiled (approx. 4.2 oz)

Calories	53
Protein	2.8 gm
Carbohydrate	12.4 gm
Fat	0.2 gm
Cholesterol	0 mg
Dietary Fiber	2.4 gm

	Amount	RDA
Folacin	53.4 mg	27%
Vitamin C	8.9 mg	15%
Magnesium	47 mg	12%
Iron	1.6 mg	11%
Potassium	316 mg	N/A

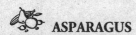 **ASPARAGUS**

Thanks to its prized culinary and medicinal properties, asparagus was beloved by the ancient Greeks and Romans alike, and was known as the ''king of vegetables.'' In days of old, in both the Western and Eastern worlds, it was used to treat a variety of common ailments, including toothaches, arthritis, bee stings and infertility.

Asparagus' Healing Properties

Although it is not known to act as a medicine against specific diseases, asparagus is nevertheless a valued member of the nutritional pharmacopoeia. A single serving contains almost half the RDA for folic acid, over one-third of the RDA for vitamin C, plus smaller amounts of potassium, beta-carotene, and other nutrients.

The most interesting new finding about asparagus is that it contains a powerful antioxidant called glutathione, which helps to fight cancer, keep men's sperm healthy, guard against cataract and heart disease, and slow the appearance and the signs of aging. Glutathione's antioxidant properties are mirrored by vitamin C, another powerful natural substance which controls oxidation.

Including the Food in Your Diet

Making asparagus a regular part of your daily diet will help to keep your body's nutrient levels high. It will also supply you with antioxidants to join in the fight against cataracts and killers such as heart disease and cancer.

Caution: *Asparagus contains substances called purines, which may be linked to the onset of gout. If you have gout, or a history of gout in your family, discuss with your physician the advisability of eating asparagus.*

ASPARAGUS
½ cup, raw

Calories	15	
Protein	2.1 gm	
Carbohydrate	2.5 gm	
Fat	0.1 gm	
Cholesterol	0 mg	
Dietary Fiber	0.7 gm	

	Amount	RDA
Folacin	95 mcg	48%
Vitamin C	22.1 mg	37%
Vitamin A	60 RE	6%
Vitamin B6	0.1 mg	5%
Iron	0.4 mg	3%
Potassium	218 mg	NA

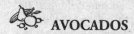 **AVOCADOS**

The avocado is native to Central America, where it has been grown for some seven thousand years. Sometimes called the "butter pear" because of the buttery texture of its fruit, the avocado was brought to North America in the 1800s. Here in the United States we primarily eat two varieties: The California avocado, which has a smooth skin, and the Florida avocado, also known as the "alligator pear" because its skin is tough and wrinkled.

The Avocado's Healing Properties

Although both experts and others have sometimes shied away from avocados because of their extremely high fat content, avocados may:

- Lower cholesterol
- Help to control damage to arteries caused by LDL ("bad") cholesterol
- Encourage arteries to open wide
- Guard against cancer

Avocados contain excellent amounts of folic acid, and very good amounts of vitamin C, thiamine, niacin, and B_6. And ounce for ounce, they have more potassium than bananas.

What Scientists Have Learned About the Avocado

Avocado and the Heart: Researchers have noted that people living in the Mediterranean area eat high-fat diets but tend to have very little heart disease. This is because a large amount of the fat that they eat comes from olive oil (rather than from meat and/or milk products, as is the case in the United States).

Most of the fat in olive oil is monounsaturated fat, a type that actually lowers bad cholesterol while leaving the good cholesterol untouched. And, acting as an antioxidant, the monounsaturated fat guards against the oxidation of LDL. (Oxidized LDL is more likely to damage artery walls.)

Although avocados are quite high in fat, most of it (about

80 percent) is monounsaturated fat. That's more monounsaturated fat than is found in olive oil, almonds, or canola oil. Australian researchers compared an avocado-rich diet (between ½ and 1½ avocados per day) to a low-fat diet. The avocado-rich diet lowered cholesterol by slightly more than 8 percent, compared to a fall of under 5 percent for the low-fat diet.

Not only do avocados help to lower cholesterol and LDL, they also act as mild vasodilators. This means that they relax the muscles surrounding the blood vessels. This, in turn, allows the vessels to open a little wider, allowing the blood to flow more freely, and blood pressure to drop.

Avocado, Sperm, Vision, and Cancer: Avocados also contain glutathione, an antioxidant that helps protect men's sperm against oxidation damage, and both sexes' eyes against oxidation-induced cataracts. Glutathione is also known to halt over twenty different cancer-causing substances, preventing the transformation of healthy cells into deadly cancerous ones.

Including the Food in Your Diet

Rotating avocados with other fruits to make up the five or more recommended servings of fruits and vegetables a day will add good amounts of potassium and other nutrients to your diet.

AVOCADO
1 (approx. 6 oz)

Calories	330
Protein	4.9 gm
Carbohydrate	27.1 gm
Fat	27 gm
Cholesterol	0 mg
Dietary Fiber	——

	Amount	RDA
Folacin	161.9 mcg	81%
Vitamin B$_6$	.9 mg	45%
Vitamin C	24 gm	40%
Niacin	5.9 mg	30%
Thiamin	.4 mg	27%
Magnesium	104 mg	26%
Riboflavin	.4 mg	22%
Vitamin A	186 RE	19%
Iron	1.6 mg	11%
Potassium	1,484 mg	NA

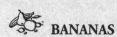 **BANANAS**

One of the first fruits to be cultivated by man, the banana remains popular today. Food historians believe that Spanish priests brought the banana to Central and South America in the 1500s. It later made its way into North America and today, the average American consumes about 25 pounds of bananas per year. (Plantains, which look like large, green bananas, are starchy relatives of the banana with similar nutritional profiles.)

The Banana's Healing Properties

One banana provides 35 percent of the RDA for vitamin B$_6$, 18 percent of the RDA for vitamin C, as well as potassium, folic acid, riboflavin, and carbohydrates. Thanks to these and other nutrients, bananas may aid in:

- Guarding against ulcers
- Preventing high blood pressure
- Preventing potentially fatal heart irregularities
- Reducing the risk of stroke
- Lowering cholesterol
- Helping to overcome insomnia

In addition, bananas have antibacterial activity, and might assist the body in resisting infection.

What Scientists Have Learned About the Banana

Bananas and Ulcers: Although bananas have been part of the diet in various parts of the world for thousands of years, it was not until the 1930s that reports on the banana's ability to treat ulcers began appearing in the medical literature. In one such study, British researchers fed bananas to laboratory mice, then gave them injections of ulcer-producing substances. Something in the bananas evidently protected the mice, for they developed relatively few ulcers.

Later research showed that bananas protect the stomach lining from stomach acids. When laboratory rats are fed aspirin, their stomach linings thin out and become more susceptible to ulcers. When the same animals are fed banana powder, their stomach linings grow thicker and stronger. Even if they are simultaneously given aspirin, banana powder helps to keep the animal's stomachs thick and strong.

Bananas and Blood Pressure: Although excess sodium (salt) is often blamed for elevating blood pressure, a relative lack of potassium can also push the pressure up. Some researchers now feel that the balance between sodium and potassium is more important than the absolute amount of sodium. This makes bananas and other potassium-rich foods good counterbalances to the typical high-sodium, low-potassium American diet.

In landmark research on potassium, researchers studied two Japanese villages. Despite the fact that the people in the villages got similar amounts of sodium from their diets, their average blood pressures were quite different. This puzzled the researchers until they realized that the villagers with the lower blood pressures were eating diets high in potassium. They realized that even if the diet is high in salt, good amounts of potassium can keep blood pressure under control by counterbalancing the sodium.

High in potassium, low in sodium, bananas help to prevent hypertension (elevated blood pressure). Doctors may also prescribe bananas when patients are put on thiazide-type blood pressure medications, such as Apresoline, Diuril, and Rauzide, which deplete the body's stores of potassium.

Bananas, the Heart, and Stroke: The potassium in bananas helps to prevent potentially dangerous heartbeats (arrhythmias) by regulating the heart's rhythm, and reduces the risk of deadly strokes as well. In a 12-year study of over 800 men and women, it was found that eating one extra helping of a potassium-rich fruit or vegetable a day lowered the risk of dying of a stroke by 40 percent.

Bananas and Cholesterol: Bananas contain pectin, a soluble fiber which helps to lower total cholesterol and LDL ("bad") cholesterol. A medium-sized banana contains about as much pectin as a medium-sized apple.

Bananas and Insomnia: Difficulty in falling or staying asleep, and/or waking too early in the morning are often symptoms of insomnia, the most common sleep disorder. Insomnia has many causes, including anxiety, depression, erratic work hours, chronic pain, and certain medications. Insomnia may also be caused by a deficiency of either niacin or vitamin B_6.

In many cases, the problem is helped by eating foods rich in tryptophan shortly before going to bed. The body converts tryptophan, a naturally occurring amino acid, into a sleep-inducing neurotransmitter called serotonin. Bananas, which contain tryptophan, are nature's sleep aids.

Including the Food in Your Diet

Regularly making a banana part of your daily fruit intake will go a long way toward protecting you against high blood pressure, irregular heartbeat, elevated cholesterol, stroke, ulcers, and insomnia. Research shows that adding even one banana to the daily diet can reduce the risk of dying of a stroke by up to 40 percent.

BANANA
1 raw (approx. 4 oz)

Calories	105	
Protein	1.2 gm	
Carbohydrate	26.8 gm	
Fat	0.6 gm	
Cholesterol	0 mg	
Dietary Fiber	1.6 gm	

	Amount	RDA
Vitamin B_6	.7 mg	35%
Vitamin C	10.3 mg	18%
Folacin	21.8 mcg	11%
Riboflavin	.2 mg	11%
Potassium	451 mg	NA

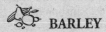 **BARLEY**

Excavations of Stone Age villages have found the remnants of barley cakes, proving that barley has been enjoyed by mankind since before the dawn of recorded history.

Barley was the basis of the diet for the ancient Roman armies who conquered much of the known world. Middle Easterners have long considered barley to be a medicine for the heart. Today, barley is one of the most important cereal crops in the world, partially because barley is used to make beer.

Barley's Healing Properties

Although barley's ample supplies of soluble and insoluble fiber are usually given credit for its medicinal prowess, the grain also contains tocotrienol and various other nutrients with important roles in promoting health. Low in fat and containing no cholesterol, barley helps to:

- Lower cholesterol
- Reduce the risk of heart disease
- Lower the incidence of stroke
- Hold cancer at bay
- Relieve constipation

What Scientists Have Learned About Barley

Barley, Cholesterol, Heart Disease, and Stroke: Barley's ability to lower cholesterol was demonstrated in American and Australian studies. In the American study, conducted at Montana State University, people on a high-barley diet enjoyed a 12 percent drop in cholesterol. In the Australian study, a barley-enhanced diet led to a 6 percent drop. Even barley oil, taken as capsules, has reduced cholesterol up to 18 percent in patients with serious heart disease.

The U.S. Department of Agriculture has devised a food additive called Oatrim, which contains the fibers found in barley and oats. Volunteers with slightly elevated cholesterol who added Oatrim to their diets saw their LDL ("bad") cholesterol fall—and they lost 4 to 5 pounds apiece, without cutting their calories.

Although the soluble fiber in barley is generally considered to be the agent responsible for lowering cholesterol, a substance found in barley (and other grains) called *tocotrienol* may also help to keep it down by interfering with the liver's ability to manufacture cholesterol.

Barley and Cancer: Barley is high in fiber, and a high-fiber diet has long been associated with a lower incidence of cancer of the colon, breast, rectum, pancreas, and prostate. Other substances in barley, called protease inhibitors, are believed to help stop cancer before it starts by preventing cancer-causing agents from harming cells of the intestinal walls.

Barley and Constipation: Constipation and irregularity are common problems for the average American consuming the typical low-fiber, high-fat diet. Fortunately, researchers in Israel have shown that eating as few as three or four barley muffins a day can relieve constipation and ensure regular bowel movements in those whose distress was so severe that they were dependent on laxatives.

Including the Food in Your Diet

The Food & Nutrition Board recommends eating six or more servings of high complex carbohydrate foods, such as grains, bread, peas, and beans, per day. A bowl of barley in the morning, or using barley instead of rice in many recipes, can help to reduce your risk of heart disease, cancer, constipation, and other ailments.

Most of the barley found in supermarkets is pearled barley. The heavily refined and scrubbed pearled barley has lost its husk and bran, along with many of its health-giving nutrients. Scotch barley is less refined, and hence more health-giving. Better still is hulled barley, which has had only its outer, inedible hull removed. Hulled barley, which is brown, contains more fiber, B-vitamins, iron, and trace minerals than the more popular pearled barley.

BARLEY, PEARLED
½ cup, cooked

Calories	97	
Protein	1.8 gm	
Carbohydrate	22.3 gm	
Fat	0.4 gm	
Cholesterol	0 mg	
Dietary Fiber	4.4 gm	

	Amount	RDA
Niacin	1.6 mg	8%
Iron	1.1 mg	7%
Folacin	12.6 mcg	6%

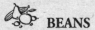 **BEANS**

Beans have been eaten by people the world over for thousands of years. During the Middle Ages, beans were such an important part of the diet in some parts of Europe that the punishment for stealing them was death. But even though the English of centuries past ate beans and used them to treat smallpox, they feared that sleeping in a bean field would drive them insane.

Like their "cousins," peas and lentils, beans are legumes, seeds filled with all the nutrients a new plant needs to grow. Many types of beans are popular today, including green beans and other "fresh beans," as well as dried beans such as navy beans, pink beans, and pinto beans.

Beans' Healing Properties

Thanks to their fiber, folic acid, iron, magnesium, zinc, and other vital nutrients, beans help to:

- Fight cancer
- Lower bad cholesterol
- Guard against heartburn
- Reduce constipation
- Keep blood sugar under control

What Scientists Have Learned About Beans

Beans and Cancer: Beans contain cancer-fighting phytoestrogens, lignans, protease inhibitors, and fiber. Phytoestrogens help to curtail the cancer-causing activity of estrogen. Lignans, which are both antioxidants and deactivators of estrogen, slow the growth of certain tumors. Protease inhibitors help cells resist cancer by keeping their DNA intact. Fiber helps to protect against several cancers. Studies have shown that people who eat large amounts of beans are less likely to develop breast cancer and less likely to succumb to cancer of the pancreas.

Beans and Heart Disease: James Anderson, M.D., of the University of Kentucky has done a great deal of research on beans and heart disease. He has found that adding a cup of cooked dried beans to the daily diet can push the LDL cholesterol down by as much as 20 percent. Eating beans also lowers the total cholesterol while raising the HDL cholesterol.

Beans, the Stomach, the Bowels, and the Blood: By neutralizing stomach acid, dried red and white beans help to prevent upset stomach and the heartburn that may result if stomach acid "splashes up" into the esophagus.

The large amounts of fiber in beans help to make the stool watery and bulky. This, in turn, allows the stool to move quickly through the bowels and exit the body easily, without the straining that encourages hemorrhoids and other problems.

Because beans release their sugar slowly into the bloodstream, they do not cause a rapid, dramatic rise in blood sugar. By helping to keep the blood sugar "level" and under control, eating beans can help certain diabetics to reduce or even eliminate their insulin injections.

Including the Food in Your Diet

One-half to one cup of cooked beans daily can reduce cholesterol by up to 10 percent in many people, and will increase the resistance to cancer and heart disease.

There are many ways to add beans to the diet. They can be eaten cooked or sprouted, or added to salads and soups. They can be made into low-fat bean dips, mashed and mixed with seasonings then spread on tacos or pitas, or made into healthful vegetarian chilies.

Beans are, unfortunately, notorious for their ability to produce intestinal gas. Saint Jerome, an early Church father, frowned on the eating of beans for he feared that the inevitable flatulence would stimulate one's private parts. In the 1960s, NASA was quite worried about the astronauts asphyxiating on their own gas in the close confines of a space capsule. One space scientist suggested that only men "who do not normally produce very large quantities of flatus" should be allowed into space.

Fortunately, rinsing, then soaking beans in water for up to an hour before cooking significantly reduces gas formation in the intestines. Adding garlic or ginger to beans also helps.

BLACK BEANS
½ cup, cooked

Calories	98	
Protein	6.4 gm	
Carbohydrate	17.7 gm	
Fat	0.4 gm	
Cholesterol	0 mg	
Dietary Fiber	4.4 gm	

	Amount	RDA
Folacin	64.2 mcg	32%
Magnesium	51.6 mg	13%
Potassium	270.2 mg	NA

KIDNEY BEANS, RED
½ cup, cooked

Calories	103	
Protein	6.8 gm	
Carbohydrate	18.7 gm	
Fat	0.4 gm	
Cholesterol	0 mg	
Dietary Fiber	4.6 gm	

	Amount	RDA
Folacin	113.7 mcg	57%
Iron	2.0 mg	13%
Magnesium	42.6 mg	11%

NAVY BEANS
½ cup, cooked

Calories	129	
Protein	7.9 gm	
Carbohydrate	23.9 gm	
Fat	0.5 gm	
Cholesterol	0 mg	
Dietary Fiber	4.9 gm	
	Amount	RDA
Folacin	127.3 mcg	64%
Iron	2.3 mg	15%
Magnesium	53.7	13%

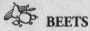 **BEETS**

Descended from chard, beets were cultivated by the Romans, who used beetroot potions to treat headaches, toothaches, and other ailments. Victorious Roman soldiers brought red and white beets to many parts of Europe, including the British Isles. Cooks in Elizabethan England had a very interesting recipe for beets, which suggested spreading a little bit of fresh dung on the beets before cooking.

The Beet's Healing Properties

Although among the sweetest-tasting of vegetables, beets are low in calories. They contain good amounts of folic acid as well as fiber, magnesium, vitamin C, potassium, and iron.

One-half cup of sliced, cooked beets provides 23 percent of the RDA for folic acid. This vitamin helps to keep the immune system strong, regulates cell division, and may help to protect women from cervical cancer. Lack of folic acid can lead to anemia, problems with digestion, malnutrition, weakness, forgetfulness, diarrhea, vomiting, poor growth in children, and birth defects. The fiber in beets helps to keep blood sugar under control, while protecting against cancers of the colon, rectum, pancreas, prostate and breast.

Including the Food in Your Diet

The Food & Nutrition Board suggests eating five or more servings of vegetables and fruits per day. Eating beets several times a week will help to protect your heart, strengthen your immune system, and increase your resistance to a variety of diseases.

BEETS		
½ cup cooked slices		
Calories	26	
Protein	0.9 gm	
Carbohydrate	5.7 gm	
Fat	0.0 gm	
Cholesterol	0 mg	
Dietary Fiber	1.4 gm	
	Amount	RDA
Folacin	45.2 mcg	23%
Magnesium	31 mg	8%
Vitamin C	4.7 mg	8%
Iron	0.5 mg	3%
Potassium	265 mg	NA

 BLUEBERRIES

Native Americans enjoyed these wild-growing berries; the Pilgrims and later immigrants also developed a taste for blueberries. These small, round berries are a superior source of vitamin C—one cup of raw blueberries contains 315 percent of the RDA for this important vitamin. They also contain fiber but are low in calories and fat.

The Blueberry's Healing Properties

This undervalued berry has many health-building properties. It helps to:

- Fight off bladder infections
- Treat diarrhea
- Reduce the risk of heart disease
- Preserve vision

Blueberries also contain a natural, aspirin-like substance. This is an interesting avenue for further investigation. In the future, will we be eating blueberries or taking "blueberry pills" to help relieve mild pain?

What Scientists Have Learned About Blueberries

Blueberries and the Bladder: Blueberries and cranberries contain substances that prevent the *E. coli* bacteria from attaching itself to the bladder wall. Unable to gain a foothold, the bacteria is simply washed away in the urine, and the bladder remains healthy.

Blueberries and Diarrhea: Blueberries, often in the form of soup made from dried blueberries, have long been used to treat diarrhea in Sweden and other countries. Modern research techniques have isolated the anti-diarrhea ingredient in blueberries: anthocyanosides, which kill *E. coli* and other organisms that can cause intestinal distress.

Blueberries and Heart Disease: Blueberries are also high in pectin fiber, which helps to lower total cholesterol and LDL ("bad") cholesterol. The fruit's anthocyanosides help to protect blood vessels from the damage caused by high cholesterol diets. Back in 1977, researchers learned that taking anthocyanosides helped patients who were suffering from diseases in which the capillaries become fragile, such as varicose veins and ulcerative dermatitis. With their ability to help keep cholesterol under control, and to prevent cholesterol-induced damage to the lining of the coronary arteries, blueberries are powerful protectors of the heart.

Blueberries and Vision: The tiny center part of the retina, called the macula, slowly deteriorates through the years under the assault of free radicals. New studies have shown that extracts made of blueberries, which not only contain high levels of anthocyanosides but also enormous amounts of the free radical quenching vitamin C, slow the loss of vision by protecting the macula.

Including the Food in Your Diet

For several months of the year, blueberries can be part of your daily fruit and vegetable intake. Eat them plain, with a fruit salad, or in muffins. They'll help keep bladder infections at bay, protect your eyes, and keep both your cholesterol and blood pressure levels down.

BLUEBERRIES
1 cup, raw

Calories	82	
Protein	1 gm	
Carbohydrate	20.5 gm	
Fat	.6 gm	
Cholesterol	0 mg	
Dietary Fiber	3.3 gm	

	Amount	RDA
Vitamin C	189 mg	315%
Potassium	129 mg	NA

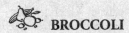 **BROCCOLI**

Descended from cabbage, broccoli was beloved by the ancient Romans, who called it "the five fingers of Jupiter." Although most modern broccoli is green, in times past purple, red, brown, and cream-colored varieties were popular.

Broccoli's Healing Properties

Considered to be a powerful cancer-fighting and immune-boosting food, broccoli is an excellent source of vitamin C, and a very good source of folacin. It also contains the cancer-fighting beta-carotene and indoles, fiber, potassium, folic acid, calcium, and selenium. Broccoli may:

- Fight cancer
- Protect against heart attacks and strokes
- Prevent constipation
- Help to control diabetes

Eating crucifers such as broccoli may also help to reduce the incidence of fibrocystic breast disease—those small, non-cancerous, sometimes painful lumps in the breast.

What Scientists Have Learned About Broccoli

Broccoli and Cancer: As stated above, broccoli is a crucifer, a member of the cruciferate family of vegetables. The cancer-fighting properties of broccoli and other crucifers have been recognized by the National Academy of Science's Committee on Diet, Nutrition and Cancer, which has stated that there is "sufficient epidemiological evidence to suggest that consumption of certain vegetables, especially . . . cruciferous vegetables . . . is associated with a reduction in the incidence of cancer at several sites in humans."

Part of broccoli's anticancer abilities comes from indoles, substances that can "turn off" the estrogen hormones which may encourage the growth of tumors (especially breast tumors). Broccoli also contains sulforaphane, an immune-boosting substance that prompts body cells to produce enzymes that fight cancer.

Antioxidants give broccoli a second way in which to fight cancer. Just ½ cup of chopped, cooked broccoli contains 82% of the RDA for vitamin C, a powerful antioxidant that helps to control the initiation and promotion of cancers in various parts of the body. Two other antioxidants in broccoli, beta-carotene and selenium, work with the C to ward off cancer.

The good amounts of fiber found in broccoli also help the

body resist cancer. Studies published over twenty years ago revealed that people who frequently ate high-fiber foods (such as broccoli and cabbage) were less likely to develop cancer of the colon. Other more recent studies support these findings, specifically pointing to raw broccoli, cabbage, and Brussels sprouts as powerful protectors against colon cancer.

Still another cancer-fighter in broccoli is chlorophyll. Chlorophyll, which gives broccoli its green color, is a proven antimutagen that guards against the alternation of cellular DNA. In addition, broccoli contains glutathione, glucosinolates, dithiolthiones, carotenoids, and other substances which make it a powerful shield against cancers of the colon, stomach, lung, prostate, larynx and esophagus.

Broccoli, Heart Disease, and Stroke: Although medical scientists have known for decades that an elevated LDL cholesterol increases the risk of heart disease, they were puzzled by the fact that not everyone with high LDLs suffered heart attacks. Upon further study, they realized that people who ate large amounts of fruits or vegetables seemed to have some protection against heart disease, even if their LDLs were high.

One of the reasons for these puzzling findings is that the LDL is more likely to leave cholesterol on artery walls if it has been oxidized. Since the vitamin C, beta-carotene, selenium, quercetin, glutathione, indoles, and lutein in broccoli are all antioxidants, eating broccoli helps to keep LDL in its less dangerous (unoxidized) state.

Broccoli, Fiber, Constipation, and Diabetes: Broccoli is a rich source of fiber. High-fiber diets guard against constipation by promoting the rapid transit of fecal matter through the bowels. And because the fiber-rich stool is softer and bulkier, it is easier to eliminate. Straining is less likely, so the risk of hemorrhoids is reduced. The fiber in broccoli also helps to slow the release of glucose (sugar) into the bloodstream after meals. This reduces the risk of diabetes, as well as subsequent diabetic damage to the heart, eyes, blood vessels, and other parts of the body. The mineral chromium in broccoli also plays a role in regulating blood sugar and insulin.

Including the Food in Your Diet

In salads, as a finger food, steamed, or as part of casseroles and other dishes, broccoli should be a frequent visitor to your lunch and dinner plates. Filled with substances that fight cancer and heart disease, tasty and easy to prepare, broccoli should be eaten several times a week or more.

BROCCOLI
½ cup, chopped, cooked

Calories	23	
Protein	2.3 gm	
Carbohydrate	4.3 gm	
Fat	0.2 gm	
Cholesterol	0 mg	
Dietary Fiber	2.0 gm	
	Amount	RDA
Vitamin C	49 mg	82%
Folacin	53.3 mcg	27%
Vitamin A	110 RE	11%
Vitamin B$_6$	0.2 mg	10%
Iron	0.9 mg	6%
Potassium	127 mg	NA

 BRUSSELS SPROUTS

Offshoots of cabbage, Brussels sprouts were developed in Belgium several hundred years ago, and were named for that country's capital, Brussels. Some botanists, however, argue that the Romans grew an early form of the cabbage cousin, and that it was eaten as a brain food. Brussels sprouts are crucifers, members of the cancer-fighting family that includes broccoli, cauliflower, cabbage, and watercress.

Brussels Sprouts' Healing Properties

Brussels sprouts are excellent sources of the antioxidant vitamin C. They also contain good amounts of folacin, plus the cancer-fighting indoles iron, potassium, and beta-carotene. Brussels sprouts may:

- Assist in the fight against cancer
- Strengthen the immune system
- Help to reduce the incidence of fibrocystic breast disease

What Scientists Have Learned About Brussels Sprouts

Brussels Sprouts and Cancer: Brussels sprouts contain several anticancer substances, including the sulforaphane which guards certain protective enzymes from being damaged by carcinogens. The indoles in Brussels sprouts lower the production of the estrogen hormones that may encourage the growth of tumors (especially breast tumors).

The glucosinolates found in Brussels sprouts demonstrated their ability to protect against cancer in an interesting study conducted at Cornell University. Researchers fed Brussels sprouts to one group of laboratory animals, glucosinolates to a second group, and nothing to a final group. All three groups were then exposed to aflatoxin, a powerful and dangerous mold associated with liver cancer and other malignancies. The animals given nothing developed liver cancer, as expected. But the animals given either the Brussels sprouts or the glucosinolates enjoyed an extra measure of protection against the cancer.

Brussels sprouts also contain chlorophyll, dithiolthiones, and other cancer-fighting substances, making it a powerful dietary tool against various forms of cancer. Just ½ cup of Brussels sprouts contains 81 percent of the RDA for vitamin C, which, like the beta-carotene in the vegetable, is a cancer-fighting antioxidant. A 1990 review article in the *Journal of the National Cancer Institute* which summarized 12 case-controlled studies, reported that simply increasing vitamin C intake could lower the incidence of breast cancer in the United States by 16 percent.

The same ½ cup of Brussels sprouts supplies over 20 percent of the RDA for folic acid. This important B-vitamin helps to prevent cancers of the rectum and cervix, as well as anemia, constipation, insomnia, weakness, headaches, memory impairment, digestive disturbances, and other ailments. The fiber in Brussels sprouts offers additional protection against cancers of the colon, rectum, pancreas, prostate, and breast.

Brussels Sprouts and Immunity: A healthy immune system is fueled by many nutrients, including the vitamin C, folic acid, iron, and beta-carotene found in Brussels sprouts. Vitamin C stimulates the immune system's T-cells and B-cells, as well as the macrophages that engulf and destroy bacteria, viruses, and other "germs." Beta-carotene, which is transformed into vitamin A in the body, enhances the activity of the natural killer cells that engage invaders in "hand-to-hand" combat. Folic acid helps the young immune-system cells to mature into full-fledged defenders of the body. And without enough iron, the numbers of T-cells and B-cells may decrease, and the lymph glands may shrivel. Together, these nutrients energize the immune system, reducing the risk of contracting anything from colds to cancer.

Including the Food in Your Diet

Brussels sprouts should be a regular addition to your plate. Even a small daily portion will help to reduce the risk of cancer and other diseases.

BRUSSELS SPROUTS
½ **cup, boiled**

Calories	30	
Protein	2.0 gm	
Carbohydrate	6.8 gm	
Fat	0.4 gm	
Cholesterol	0 mg	
Dietary Fiber	3.4 gm	
	Amount	RDA
Vitamin C	48.4 mg	81%
Folacin	46.8 mcg	23%
Iron	0.9 mg	6%
Potassium	247.3 mg	NA

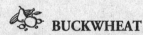 **BUCKWHEAT**

Not a wheat at all, or even a grain, buckwheat is the fruit of a leafy plant native to Asia, and is related to rhubarb. Buckwheat is usually cooked and served like rice, or used to make flour which is then used to make pancakes. Kasha is a popular form of roasted and cracked buckwheat kernels.

Buckwheat's Healing Properties

Buckwheat contains fiber, magnesium, and an amino acid named lysine. Thanks to the lysine, buckwheat may help to reduce the severity and frequency of herpes, shingles, and Epstein-Barr (EB) virus. These three diseases thrive in the presence of another amino acid, called arginine. Lysine acts as an arginine antagonist, balancing out or "neutralizing" arginine's effects. Studies have shown that low levels of lysine in the blood put one at risk for herpes, and that giving lysine supplements can reduce the frequency and severity of herpes attacks.

In a study of 52 herpes simplex patients suffering from recurrent oral infections, genital infections, or both, some were given lysine and others a placebo. The patients were also told to avoid nuts, chocolate, and gelatin, which are high in arginine. After six months, the lysine group had fewer herpes outbreaks, and the ones they did have were milder.

In addition to lysine's anti-herpes, shingles, and EB virus effects, buckwheat contains fiber to help reduce constipation and control blood sugar. And since it contains no wheat, buckwheat is a good dietary alternative for those who are allergic to wheat.

Including the Food in Your Diet

Although not a grain, buckwheat (or kasha) is an excellent substitute for rice in main dishes, or as a side dish. Sprinkled with a dash of cinnamon, it makes an excellent breakfast cereal. Enjoying buckwheat several times a week is a tasty way to improve general health.

BUCKWHEAT GROATS
½ cup, cooked

Calories	91	
Protein	3.4 gm	
Carbohydrate	19.7 gm	
Fat	0.6 gm	
Cholesterol	0 mg	
Dietary Fiber	——	

	Amount	RDA
Magnesium	50.5 mg	13%
Folacin	13.9 mcg	7%
Iron	0.8 mg	5%

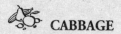 **CABBAGE**

Cabbage has been cultivated and eaten for thousands of years. The ancient Romans used the vegetable to treat wounds, cancer, colic, paralysis, and drunkenness, and to prevent the plague. They also considered it to be quite tasty: The Emperor Claudius is said to have asked the Roman Senate to vote as to whether or not cabbage and corned beef was the best-tasting dinner ever devised. (The Senators unanimously voted ''yes.'')

Caesar's Roman legions brought cabbage with them to England, and by the sixteenth century the vegetable was felt to be useful in treating bruises, poisoning, deafness, dog bites, and acne. Cabbage was used well into the twentieth century to treat asthma, cancer, gangrene, tuberculosis, and other serious diseases. Today we know that cabbage is a crucifer. The crucifers, more properly known as the cruciferous family of vegetables, are so named because their leaves grow at right angles to each other, forming a cross (crucifer). The crucifers contain many cancer-fighting substances, including sulforaphane, indoles, beta-carotene, vitamin C, and fiber. Other members of the crucifer family include broccoli, cauliflower, and Brussels sprouts.

Cabbage's Healing Properties

Chinese cabbage is a tremendous source of vitamin C, with ½ cup of shredded Chinese cabbage providing over 360 percent of the RDA for this vitamin. The more common red and green cabbage are good sources of C, offering 20 to 40 percent of the RDA for the vitamin. Cabbage also contains fiber, B-vitamins, and other nutrients. Among its many health-promoting properties, cabbage may:

• Reduce the risk of cancer
• Be useful in treating ulcers
• Have antibacterial and antiviral properties

Eating cabbage and other crucifers may also help to reduce the incidence of fibrocystic breast disease (small, noncancerous, possibly painful lumps in the breast). Various nutrients in cabbage stimulate the immune system, while cabbage's fiber promotes regularity and reduces the risk of hemorrhoids and other ailments associated with constipation.

What Scientists Have Learned About Cabbage

Cabbage and Cancer: Cabbage contains chlorophyll, dithiolthiones, flavonoids, isothiocyantes, phenols, and other factors that make it a strong shield against cancers of the colon and rectum. Cabbage also contains indoles, substances that can slow the production of the estrogens which can encourage the growth of breast and other tumors.

Cabbage's vitamin C serves as an antioxidant, helping to control the oxidants and free radicals that damage cells and encourage cancer. The fiber in cabbage is another anticancer factor. People who frequently eat raw cabbage, broccoli, and Brussels sprouts and other high-fiber foods are less likely to develop cancer of the colon. Indeed, research has shown that eating cabbage two or more times a week reduces the odds of colon cancer in men by 66 percent. Other studies have demonstrated cabbage's ability to protect against cancers of the stomach and lungs.

Cabbage and Ulcers: Beginning back in the 1940s, studies have shown that drinking large amounts of cabbage juice (up to a quart a day) may help to cure intestinal ulcers. The development of powerful ulcer medications swept aside the notion of drinking cabbage juice until 1973, when it was discovered that certain constituents of ulcer drugs were identical to substances found in cabbage.

Another explanation for the ability of cabbage to treat ulcers may lie in the fact that cabbage has antibiotic properties. Cabbage may fight ulcers by attacking the bacteria that we have only recently realized may cause ulcers. Although eating cabbage has not yet replaced medication as a cure for ulcers, adding large amounts of cabbage to the diet may be a prudent measure for those concerned about preventing the painful intestinal disorder.

Cabbage and Infections: Laboratory studies have shown that cabbage deactivates viruses and bacteria, possibly by stimulating the immune system to produce more antibodies against these invading organisms.

Including the Food in Your Diet

As little as two tablespoons of cooked cabbage a day have been shown to lower the risk of stomach cancer. As stated above, two or more servings a week have lowered the risk of colon cancer in men by up to 66 percent. Making cabbage part of your daily diet, or at least having several servings per week, will help to hold cancer and other diseases at bay.

Red cabbage, green cabbage, Savoy cabbage, Bok choy (Chinese cabbage), and Napa cabbage all have healing properties. Raw cabbage has figured prominently in many cabbage cancer studies, and some of cabbage's healing substances are damaged by heat, so it's best to eat at least some of your daily cabbage raw. Coleslaw, a cabbage salad, has also been found to have anticancer properties.

COMMON (GREEN) CABBAGE
½ cup shredded, cooked

Calories	16	
Protein	0.7 gm	
Carbohydrate	3.6 gm	
Fat	0.2 gm	
Cholesterol	0 mg	
Dietary Fiber	1.8 gm	

	Amount	RDA
Vitamin C	18.2 mg	30%
Folacin	15.2 mcg	8%

Red cabbage has more vitamin C than common cabbage, and is a good source of vitamin B_6.

```
                      RED CABBAGE
                ½ cup shredded, cooked

     Calories              16
     Protein               0.8 gm
     Carbohydrate          3.5 gm
     Fat                   0.2 gm
     Cholesterol           0   mg
     Dietary Fiber         1.8 gm

                          Amount          RDA
     Vitamin C             2.6 mg         43%
     Vitamin B₆            0.1 mg          5%
```

Savoy cabbage provides generous amounts of fiber and vitamins A and C, plus smaller amounts of vitamin B_6.

```
                     SAVOY CABBAGE
                ½ cup shredded, cooked

     Calories              18
     Protein               1.3 gm
     Carbohydrate          4.0 gm
     Fat                   0.1 gm
     Cholesterol           0   mg
     Dietary Fiber         2.3 gm

                          Amount          RDA
     Vitamin C            12.5 mg         21%
     Folacin              34   mcg        17%
     Vitamin A            65               7%
```

Bok choy, also known as Chinese cabbage, is a superb source of vitamin A. Including large amounts of Chinese cabbage in the diet may help to prevent cancer, protect the heart, lower cholesterol, and control blood sugar.

BOK CHOY (CHINESE CABBAGE)
½ cup shredded, cooked

Calories	10
Protein	1.3 gm
Carbohydrate	1.5 gm
Fat	0.1 gm
Cholesterol	0 mg
Dietary Fiber	1.4 gm

	Amount		RDA
Vitamin C	221	mg	368%
Vitamin A	218	RE	22%
Folacin	34.5	mcg	17%
Calcium	79	mg	7%
Iron	0.9	mg	6%

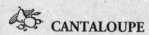 CANTALOUPE

The round fruit is named after the Italian town of Cantalupa, where it was first cultivated in Europe many hundreds of years ago. Cantalupa, which means "wolf howl," was where the popes went for a vacation from the Vatican—and apparently where wolves gathered to sing.

Cantaloupe, a member of the melon family, is related to the casaba, honeydew, crenshaw, Juan Canary, Persian, Santa Clause, and watermelon. Although popular in the ancient world, melons did not gain widespread acceptance in Northern Europe until they were introduced in France in the fifteenth century. However, melons had long been available and popular in Asia, the South Pacific, and Africa, where they were used to treat hepatitis, worms, cancer, and menstrual difficulties.

What is commonly called a "cantaloupe" is actually (botanically speaking) a muskmelon. The true cantaloupe, grown and eaten primarily in Europe, is not readily available in the United States.

The Cantaloupe's Healing Properties

Half a cantaloupe supplies 180 percent of the RDA for vitamin C, excellent amounts of beta-carotene, plus folacin, vitamin B$_6$, potassium, and fiber. Low in fat, calories, and sodium, cantaloupe may:

- Thin the blood
- Increase one's resistance to cancer
- Protect the heart

What Scientists Have Learned About the Cantaloupe

Cantaloupe and the Blood: When blood clots become wedged into already narrowed arteries in the heart and brain, they can precipitate heart attacks and strokes. Like onions and garlic, cantaloupe contains adenosine, a substance that helps to prevent the coagulation of the blood and the formation of these unwanted blood clots.

Cantaloupe and Antioxidants: Cantaloupe is an excellent source of vitamin C, with ½ of an average melon providing over 180 percent of the RDA for C, and 86 percent of the suggested daily dose of beta-carotene. Ample amounts of these two antioxidants and free radical quenchers help to strengthen the immune system, ward off cancer, lessen the risk of heart disease, reduce oxidation damage to the body, slow the signs and symptoms of aging, and keep a man's sperm healthy and vigorous.

Cantaloupe and Potassium: Cantaloupe is a rich source of potassium, a mineral that plays an important role in preventing acne, fatigue, nervousness, breathing difficulties, and certain forms of depression. Potassium is also necessary to keep the blood pressure at safe levels, and to keep the heart beating properly. Ample amounts of potassium may also help to prevent strokes.

CANTALOUPE
½ raw (approx. 9.5 oz)

Calories	95
Protein	2.5 gm
Carbohydrate	22.4 gm
Fat	0.8 gm
Cholesterol	0 mg
Dietary Fiber	0.9 gm

	Amount	RDA
Vitamin C	112.7 mg	186%
Vitamin A	861 RE	86%
Folacin	45.5 mcg	23%
Vitamin B$_6$	.4 mg	20%
Potassium	825 mg	NA

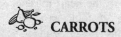 **CARROTS**

Purple carrots? Red and black carrots? The earliest carrots, scrawny and multicolored natives of Afghanistan, had none of the familiar orange color. The vegetable spread first to ancient Greece, then to Rome, and later to Europe. A pale yellow carrot first showed up in Western Europe in the 1500s, and Dutch cross-breeders developed the modern-looking orange carrot over the next century.

Through the years, carrots have been used to treat skin problems, nervousness, respiratory difficulties, and, of course, vision problems. In fact, seeking an edge over the enemy in World War II, the British fed their fighter pilots special carrots that were extra high in beta-carotene, hoping to improve their night vision.

The Carrot's Healing Properties

A single carrot contains tremendous amounts of beta-carotene, which can be converted in the body into vitamin A.

In fact, beta-carotene and the other carotenes are named for carrots, the food in which they were discovered. Carrots also provide C and B_6, folic acid, iron, and potassium. Eating carrots may:

- Lessen the odds of heart disease
- Reduce the risk of cancer
- Protect the vision well into the senior years
- Strengthen the immune system
- Fight against constipation.

What Scientists Have Learned About the Carrot

Carrots & Heart Disease: Heart disease is the number one killer disease in the United States. Although the biochemical details are complex, the general sequence of events leading to heart disease is easy to understand. Imagine that you're trying to drive home on the freeway, but you're getting nowhere; the traffic is so bad, no one can move ahead. The same general idea applies to heart disease. You want fresh blood to "drive through" your arteries, bringing oxygen to the heart muscle. But it can't get through because packets of cholesterol, fat, and cellular debris growing out from the artery walls are blocking the way. Caught in this arterial "traffic," the fresh blood can't deliver oxygen to the heart muscle, and that muscle dies. We call this death of heart muscle a heart attack. Fortunately, carrots work in several ways to prevent heart disease:

Fiber: Carrots are high in soluble fiber; eating large amounts of soluble-fiber foods can push the cholesterol levels down. Part of the fiber found in carrots is in the form of pectin, which is also known to reduce cholesterol. Carrot fiber contains calcium pectate, a substance that lowers cholesterol by binding to bile acids and preventing them from being reabsorbed into the body. According to scientists at the U.S. Department of Agriculture, if people with elevated cholesterol eat just 2 carrots a day, their cholesterol levels may fall by 10 to 20 percent.

Beta-carotene: Beta-carotene's role in preventing heart disease was scrutinized during the nationwide Physician's Health Study. As part of the study, 160 male doctors, each of whom had a history of heart disease, were given either 50 mg of beta-carotene every other day or a placebo. When the two groups were examined several years later, the one that had received beta-carotene had experienced only half the heart attacks and other heart problems than the placebo group did. The beta-carotene and other carotenes in carrots are powerful protectors of the heart.

Vitamin C: The vitamin C in carrots is known to help in the battle against heart disease in at least two ways. As an antioxidant, it controls the oxidative changes that can make LDL ("bad") cholesterol even more dangerous by making it more likely to "stick" to artery walls. And blood levels of vitamin C have been linked to the levels of beneficial HDL: The more C in the blood, the higher the protective HDL and the lower the risk of heart disease.

B_6: Although only small amounts of B_6 are found in carrots, the vitamin plays a major role in preventing heart disease. Studies with laboratory animals have shown that a lack of B_6 in the diet can lead to severe damage to the arteries. The actual arterial damage may be caused by an amino acid called homocysteine, which is normally supposed to be converted into the less dangerous cystathionine. But B_6 is necessary for the conversion, so insufficient supplies of B_6 may allow the dangerous homocysteine to build up and harm the vital arterial linings.

Fat: Carrots are also low in fat, which makes up only 4 percent of their calories. That's good for people concerned about maintaining

healthy hearts, for eating a low-fat diet can
help to reduce cholesterol.

With all these factors (fiber, beta-carotene, vitamin C, B_6,
and low fat) combined, the carrot is a powerful medicine for
the heart.

Carrots and Cancer: The same fiber, beta-carotene, vitamin
C, and lack of fat in carrots which improve heart health also
strengthen the body in its fight against cancer. High-fiber diets
have been credited with reducing the incidence of cancers of
the breast, colon, rectum, pancreas, and prostate. Diets low in
fat or animal fat have been linked to a reduced risk of breast
cancer, intestinal cancer, lung cancer, ovarian cancer and prostate cancer.

The beta-carotene in carrots is transformed into vitamin A
once inside the body. Many studies have shown that vitamin
A/beta-carotene fights off cancers of the bladder, esophagus,
stomach, larynx, lung, prostate, cervix, neck, and head. And
the vitamin C found in the orange vegetable has been credited
with staving off many of the same cancers.

Two other substances in carrots, *p*-coumaric acid and chloregenic acid, help reduce the risk of cancer by binding on to
the nitric oxides in our food. The "bound and gagged" nitric
oxides are then flushed out of the body, instead of being converted into potentially cancer-causing nitrosamines. Carrots
also contain lycopene, a powerful antioxidant that helps to
reduce the risk of several different cancers.

Carrots and the Eyes: Contrary to popular belief, eating carrots will *not* improve night vision in normal, healthy people.
However, the beta-carotene and vitamin C in carrots will help
slow the damage to vision caused by age-related macular degeneration (AMD), a disease which causes progressive deterioration of the part of the retina called the macula. Almost
everyone suffers from AMD to one degree or another as they
age.

It's felt that AMD is caused by oxidative damage to the
macula. As antioxidants, the beta-carotene and C in carrots
help to slow, or possibly halt, the progress of AMD. In fact,
information from the first National Health and Nutrition Examination Survey showed that people eating the most vege-

tables high in beta-carotene and C had the least amount of damage to the precious macula.

Including the Food in Your Diet

Eating just two carrots a day is enough to lower cholesterol in many people with elevated levels, and to bestow protection against cancer.

Eating too many carrots is not dangerous, but it may cause the skin to turn slightly yellowish. Caused by an excess of carotenoid pigments, the coloring will quickly vanish if one stops eating carrots, or consumes fewer.

CARROT
1 medium (approx. 2.5 oz)

Calories	31	
Protein	0.7 gm	
Carbohydrate	5.6 gm	
Fat	0.1 gm	
Cholesterol	0 mg	
Dietary Fiber	1.2 gm	

	Amount		RDA
Vitamin A	2025	RE	202%
Vitamin C	6.7	mg	11%
Folacin	10	mcg	5%
Potassium	233	mg	NA

 CAULIFLOWER

Although Mark Twain dismissed cauliflower as "nothing but cabbage with a college education," the white-topped vegetable has been popular for centuries, especially in France. Cauliflower contains cancer-fighting substances, but is not as nutrient-packed as other members of the cabbage family. Specifically, it hasn't as much of the chlorophyll and carotenes that give vegetables their color, as well as their ability to resist oxidation-induced damage to body cells.

Cauliflower's Healing Properties

Like other members of the crucifer family of vegetables, cauliflower contains indoles, sulforphane, and vitamin C, three powerful cancer-fighters. The indoles slow the production of estrogen hormones that may encourage the growth of tumors (especially breast tumors). Sulforaphane assists designated enzymes in protecting body cells from certain carcinogens. Just ½ cup of cooked cauliflower offers 57 percent of the RDA for vitamin C, whose antioxidant properties protect against various types of cancer. Eating cauliflower and other crucifers may also help to reduce the incidence of fibrocystic breast disease.

Including the Food in Your Diet

Cauliflower should be a regular addition to your plate. It is delicious raw in salads, as a "finger food" on vegetable platters, or steamed.

Cauliflower is often boiled or otherwise cooked for long periods of time. Extended cooking destroys key nutrients in the vegetable, so it should be cooked as little as possible. It's best to steam for a few minutes, just until tender. Raw cauliflower is also a healthy and tasty addition to any menu.

CAULIFLOWER
½ cup, cooked

	Amount	RDA
Calories	15	
Protein	1.2 gm	
Carbohydrate	2.9 gm	
Fat	0.1 gm	
Cholesterol	0 mg	
Dietary Fiber	1.0 gm	
Vitamin C	34.3 mg	57%
Folacin	31.7 mcg	16%
Potassium	200 mg	NA

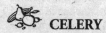 **CELERY**

Celery gum? Celery soup? Celery soda? Celery elixir sold through the Sears & Roebuck catalog as a treatment for nervous ailments? It's all true. In fact, throughout most of the 1800s, celery was considered to be an aristocratic food. Only society's finest could afford the expensive vegetable, which was served in special celery holders. Unfortunately for celery, it became inexpensive and widely available in the 1880s. Since everyone could afford to eat it, few people wanted to, and celery lost most of its great popularity.

A member of the carrot family, celery is most likely native to Eurasia. It was used in Egypt for impotence, and in ancient Rome to treat hangovers and constipation. During the Middle Ages, celery was given to people suffering from gallstones, animal bites, and constipation. France's Madame Pompadour, mistress to King Louis XV, fed her royal lover celery as an aphrodisiac.

Celery's Healing Properties

Although celery does not have "negative calories" that cause celery eaters to lose weight (as many people would like to believe), it is very low in calories. Celery may help to:

- Protect against cancer
- Reduce the risk of heart disease
- Fight infections

What Scientists Have Learned About Celery

Celery and Cancer: Celery contains phthalides, polyacetylenes, and several other substances that disarm carcinogens before they can transform normal cells into cancerous ones. Celery appears to be especially protective against stomach cancer.

Celery, Blood Pressure, Heart Disease, and Stroke: Although Western physicians have traditionally been suspicious of celery because it contains a large amount of sodium, the Chinese have used celery to control blood pressure for more than 2,000 years. We now know that celery contains a substance called 3-n-butylphthalide, which causes the smooth muscle surrounding the blood vessels to relax. Relaxed, the vessels open wider and allow blood to flow more easily, thus decreasing the blood pressure. Feeding laboratory animals each day the amount of 3-n-butylphthalide found in four celery stalks caused their blood pressure to fall by over 10 percent—and their cholesterol levels to drop, as well. Lowering blood pressure and cholesterol reduces the risk of heart attacks and stroke.

It has been theorized that celery relaxes the smooth muscles surrounding the blood vessels by interfering with stress-related hormones that would otherwise force the muscles to tighten up. If this is correct, celery's blood pressure–lowering abilities would work best in people who are under stress.

Celery and Infections: Along with cabbage, carrots, licorice, nutmeg, ginger, and onions, celery has antibacterial action, and may assist the immune system in resisting infections.

Including the Food in Your Diet

You can munch on celery as a snack, or add it to salads. Although we don't know if four stalks a day is the exact prescription for humans, it's easy to add several low-calorie celery stalks to the daily diet.

CELERY
1 stalk, raw (approx. 1.5 oz)

Calories	6
Protein	0.3 gm
Carbohydrate	1.4 gm
Fat	0.1 gm
Cholesterol	0 mg
Dietary Fiber	0.4 gm

	Amount	RDA
Vitamin C	2.5 mg	4%
Folacin	3.6 mcg	2%

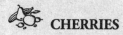 **CHERRIES**

Close cousin to the plum, the cherry is a low-fat treat that provides moderate amounts of vitamin C, plus modest portions of iron and potassium. As far back as 300 B.C., the Greeks used the cherry as a cure for epilepsy. In later eras, cherries were prescribed for kidney ailments.

The Cherry's Healing Properties

Although cherries have not traditionally been considered nutritional standouts, more recent research has highlighted the value of the flavonoids found in the small round fruit. Pigments found in plants, flavonoids protect the body against the damage caused by free radicals, and enhance the body's ability to deal with carcinogens, viruses, and other troubling substances. It appears that anthocyanidins and proanthocyanidins, two types of flavonoids found in cherries, also help move vitamin C into the body's cells, and to keep the blood-carrying capillaries and the joints strong.

Including the Food in Your Diet

Health experts recommend eating five to six servings of fruit and vegetables a day. Frequently including cherries in your daily intake when they are in season will help to keep your immune system strong.

CHERRIES, SWEET
10 raw (approx. 2.4 oz)

Calories	50	
Protein	0.9 gm	
Carbohydrate	11.3 gm	
Fat	.7 gm	
Cholesterol	0 mg	
Dietary Fiber	1.1 gm	

	Amount	RDA
Vitamin C	4.8 mg	8%
Iron	.3 mg	2%
Potassium	152 mg	NA

CHICORY

Native to India, this member of the daisy family was used in ancient Mediterranean cultures such as those of the Greeks, Romans, and Egyptians. Perhaps the first mention of chicory in Western writings occurred in 1651 when the chef to France's King Henri IV published a book of recipes that explained, among other things, how to cook chicory. Sometimes called curly endive, chicory looks like a ragged head of lettuce.

Chicory's Healing Properties

Although a relatively rare visitor to the typical dinner plate, chicory is surprisingly nutritious. Just ½ cup of chopped raw chicory supplies almost 50 percent of the RDA for folic acid, well over 30 percent of the RDA for vitamin C, plus beta-carotene, potassium, and fiber.

Folic acid plays an important but often overlooked role in preventing heart disease. Excessive amounts of an amino acid called homocysteine can damage the arteries of men and women, as well as the bones of menopausal women, leading to osteoporosis. By preventing the buildup of homeocysteine, folic acid guards the heart and the bones.

The vitamin C and beta-carotene in folic acid are antioxidants which help to prevent the oxidative damage that can lead to cancer, as well as the oxidative changes that can make LDL (''bad'') cholesterol more dangerous to arteries and the heart. Chicory's fiber guards against both cancer and constipation, while helping to keep the blood sugar and cholesterol under control.

Including the Food in Your Diet

Add chicory to your salads often. Its folacin, beta-carotene, and vitamin C will help to keep your immune system strong.

CHICORY
½ cup chopped, raw

Calories	21	
Protein	1.5 gm	
Carbohydrate	4.2 gm	
Fat	0.3 gm	
Cholesterol	0 mg	
Dietary Fiber	3.6 gm	
	Amount	RDA
Folacin	98 mcg	49%
Vitamin A	360 RE	36%
Vitamin C	21.6 mg	36%

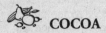 COCOA

Originating in South America, the cocoa tree spread north to Central America by the seventh century A.D., where it was enjoyed by the Aztecs, Mayans, and other cultures. Introduced by European explorers to the Old World, cocoa paste and drinks gained widespread popularity when sugar and spices such as vanilla and cinnamon were added to the bitter-tasting original recipes. Wealthy Spaniards of the 1600s loved cocoa so much that they had their servants serve it to them, fresh and hot, during church services. A bishop who frowned on this practice threatened to excommunicate anyone who drank chocolate in church. French priests didn't have a problem with worshipers sipping cocoa when they should have been praying, but they were suspicious of the dark-colored fluid, fearing that it had been concocted by evil magicians and devil-worshipers to lure unsuspecting people away from God.

Although not normally considered a "health food," an occasional cup of hot cocoa made with nonfat ("skim") milk can help to keep the immune system and the mind in tiptop shape by supplying the body with key nutrients.

Cocoa's Healing Properties

Cocoa is a good source of B-vitamins. Eight fluid ounces of hot cocoa provides nearly 45 percent of the RDA for vitamin B_{12}, and good amounts of B_1, B_2, B_6, and folic acid.

The B-vitamins play many roles in health. They help the body to draw energy out of food, keep the nerves and skin healthy, and strengthen the immune system. Vitamin B_{12} and folic acid ensure the maturation of immune-system cells in the bone marrow. Without sufficient B_{12}, the numbers of T- and B-cells will fall. A deficiency of B_6 causes the thymus gland, where the T-cells are readied for battle, to shrink. Shortages of B_2 can reduce the body's ability to produce antibodies, while a lack of B_1 can weaken the immune system in many ways. The B-family vitamins are also "medicines for the mind," helping to ward off anxiety, nervousness, depression, irritability, and personality changes.

In addition to B-vitamins, cocoa contains calcium, magnesium, iron, and zinc.

COCOA
1 cup, made with nonfat milk

Calories	148	
Protein	9.5	mg
Carbohydrate	30	mg
Fat	9	mg
Cholesterol	2	mg
Dietary Fiber	0.2	gm

	Amount		RDA
Vitamin A	150	RE	15%
Folacin	13	mcg	6%
Niacin	.2	mg	1%
Calcium	310	mg	26%
Magnesium	50	mg	12%

 COLLARD GREENS

Looking something like spinach but tasting like cabbage or kale, collard greens are members of the cancer-fighting crucifer family of vegetables. The ancient Romans prized collards because they felt that eating the vegetable would prevent one's mind from being muddled by wine.

Collard Greens' Healing Properties

Collard greens contain indoles and other substances known to increase the body's resistance to cancer. Collards also contain good amounts of beta-carotene and vitamin C, two antioxidants that help to reduce the risk of heart disease and cancer by controlling the oxidants which damage (oxidize) the lining of the arteries, cellular DNA, and other parts of the body. Both of these vitamins can also strengthen the immune system, and may delay and/or soften the symptoms of aging.

Collard's fiber helps to protect against cancer of the colon, rectum, prostate, pancreas, and breast, as well as helping with constipation.

Including the Food in Your Diet

Adding collard greens to your salads every chance you get is an easy and tasty way to bolster your general health and reduce the risk of cancer. Of course, eating them with ham hocks or other fatty foods is counterproductive, for a large load of fat can outweigh the benefits of low-fat collard greens.

COLLARD GREENS
½ cup chopped, cooked

Calories	13	
Protein	1.1 gm	
Carbohydrate	2.5 gm	
Fat	0.1 gm	
Cholesterol	0 mg	
Dietary Fiber	——	

	Amount	RDA
Vitamin A	211 RE	21%
Vitamin C	9.3 mg	16%

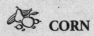 **CORN**

No one knows where corn came from. The best guess is that it originated as a wild grass in Mexico and Central America. Corn became a major part of the Colonial American diet, and corn whiskey was a popular remedy for arthritis, toothaches, coughs, colds, consumption, and various other ailments. (Its great popularity makes you wonder if corn whiskey was really that effective, or simply easier to swallow than other medicines.)

When Americans say "corn," they're referring to yellow

kernels on a cob. But in England wheat is called "corn," while "corn" means oats in Scotland. The confusion arises from that fact that the most common cereal grain in many countries or regions is often called "corn."

Corn's Healing Properties

Low in fat, corn provides complex carbohydrates and fiber, plus vitamins B_1 and C, folic acid, niacin, and magnesium.

The complex carbohydrates and fiber in corn help to keep blood sugar under control, reducing the risk of diabetes and diabetic damage to the heart, eyes, blood vessels and other parts of the body. Corn's fiber offers protection against cancers of the colon, rectum, pancreas, prostate, and breast, as well as constipation and hemorrhoids.

Including the Food in Your Diet

Eating several cobs of corn per week (when they are in season) adds tasty nutrition to your diet.

CORN, YELLOW
½ cup cut, cooked (4" ear)

	Amount	RDA
Calories	89	
Protein	2.7 gm	
Carbohydrate	20.6 gm	
Fat	1.1 gm	
Cholesterol	0 mg	
Dietary Fiber	3.0 gm	
	Amount	RDA
Folacin	38.1 mcg	19%
Thiamin	0.2 mg	13%
Vitamin C	5.1 mg	9%
Magnesium	26 mg	7%
Niacin	1.3 mg	7%
Potassium	204 mg	NA

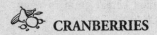 **CRANBERRIES**

Grown in Asia, Europe, and North America, cranberries were used by American Indians to speed the healing of wounds, and have a long history of use in treating urinary tract infections. Cranberries have also been ingested, whole or in juice form, or crushed and rubbed on the skin to treat fever, skin rash, and headaches.

The Cranberry's Healing Properties

With little fat and few calories, cranberries contain fiber and good amounts of vitamin C. Many studies have shown that cranberries can help to:

• Prevent urinary tract infections

What Scientists Have Learned About the Cranberry

Cranberries and Bladder Infections: Although doctors have long known that drinking cranberry juice reduces the incidence of bladder infections, they didn't know why. Their best guess was that the juice made the urine too acidic for the bacteria which caused the infections. That was a reasonable hypothesis, but it turns out that acidity is not what gives cranberries their antibacterial properties. Instead, "teflon-like" substances in cranberry juice act like grease on the bladder wall, preventing the bacteria from "grabbing hold" and causing disease.

In a landmark study of cranberries and bladder infections, Dr. Papas of Tufts University gave each of 60 patients 16 ounces of cranberry juice per day for three weeks. The juice prevented infections in over 70 percent of the volunteers, but the problems reappeared when they stopped drinking the "bladder greasing" juice.

Including the Food in Your Diet

Between 1 and 2 cups of cranberry juice a day is enough to ward off bladder infections, and possibly other urinary tract infections in those infected by susceptible organisms. Or, if you prefer, eat fresh cranberries when they are in season, either by themselves or in a fruit salad.

> **Caution:** *Since cranberries contain oxalic acid, they should be eaten with caution by those with kidney stones, or a tendency toward kidney stones. Consult your physician if there is a history of stones in your family.*

CRANBERRIES
1 cup, raw

	Amount	
Calories	46	
Protein	0.4 gm	
Carbohydrate	12.1 gm	
Fat	0.2 gm	
Cholesterol	0 mg	
Dietary Fiber	1.0 gm	

	Amount	RDA
Vitamin C	12.8 mg	21%

 CUCUMBERS

Cucumbers were gathered and possibly cultivated in Southeast Asia as far back as 9750 B.C. Despite man's long acquaintance with the watery green vegetable, timid Englishmen of the 1600s feared that eating cucumbers would lead to certain death. (They also believed that lying on a bed of the vegetables would cure fevers, and that wearing one about the waist was guaranteed to make a woman more fertile!)

The Cucumber's Healing Properties

Cucumbers are very low in fat and calories. Over 90 percent water, they contain good amounts of vitamin C, plus fiber, folic acid, and potassium. Cucumbers also contain small amounts of silica, a mineral necessary for the body to build the connective tissue which holds bone, muscle, ligaments, tendons, and cartilage together.

Including the Food in Your Diet

Although the cucumbers are not a nutritional standout, they make an excellent addition to any diet. Eating up to half a medium-sized cucumber a day, by itself or sliced into a salad, will help to round out a nutritious diet.

CUCUMBER		
1 cup, raw		
Calories	46	
Protein	0.4 gm	
Carbohydrate	12.1 gm	
Fat	0.2 gm	
Cholesterol	0 mg	
Dietary Fiber	1.0 gm	
	Amount	RDA
Vitamin C	12.8 mg	21%

 CURRANTS (Black, Red & White)

The black currant, a close relative of the berry family, has been used to treat constipation, stress, colds and other respiratory ailments. Rarely found in the fruit aisles of supermarkets, instead the currant is more likely to turn up in liqueur or preserves. That's a waste of a good berry, for the black currant is a superlative source of vitamin C. A single cup of the small black berries contains well over 300 percent of the RDA for this vitamin. Red and white currants, which contain about 77 percent of the RDA for vitamin C per cup, are usually eaten in jellies and jams.

The Currant's Healing Properties:

The amounts of vitamin C in currants give these berries many medicinal properties.

Vitamin C helps lower the total cholesterol (if it is elevated), while increasing the "good" HDL cholesterol, which protects against clogged arteries and heart disease.

In addition to shielding the heart, vitamin C "disarms" oxidants in the body. Vitamin C has specifically been credited with protecting against cancers of the esophagus, stomach, pancreas, cervix, rectum, breast, and lungs.

The currant's vitamin C also increases resistance to glaucoma and macular degeneration, two common eye ailments. Caused by an increase in fluid and pressure in the eyeball, glaucoma damages and eventually destroys vision. Researchers have found a relationship between how much vitamin C one consumes and pressure in the eyes. In an early study, a single dose of 500 mg of vitamin C per kilogram of body weight lowered pressure in the eyeballs of 39 patients. Smaller doses spread throughout the day were also effective, and less likely to cause the loose stools some people experience with large doses of vitamin C. These results were confirmed by a subsequent study of 25 senior citizens suffering from moderately high pressure in the eyeballs. After 6 days of 500 mg of vitamin C four times per day, the pressure in their eyes fell significantly.

The other common vision problem, age-related macular degeneration (AMD), results from progressive damage to the macula caused by "routine" oxidation. The large amounts of C in currants help to slow the progression of AMD by protecting the macular cells from oxidation.

The versatile vitamin C performs many other duties. Acting as an antihistamine, it may reduce the symptoms of seasonal allergic rhinitis. The vitamin has successfully been used to treat the skin disease known as eczema, which, in its later stages, is characterized by thick, crusted, scaly skin. Test tube studies have shown that vitamin C may also be able to slow the progress of AIDS (Acquired Immunodeficiency Syndrome). The symptoms of AIDS and AIDS-related complex were reduced in over 250 HIV-positive patients given 20 to 200 grams of C per day.

Currants also contain flavonoids, substances that strengthen the body's ability to resist viruses, allergens and carcinogens. Various flavonoids also strengthen the body's collagen, a protein that helps to hold cartilage, tendons, and ligaments together.

Including the Food in Your Diet

A single cup of currants a day offers a great deal of protection against heart disease, cancer, and other common ailments.

Caution: *Since currants contain oxalic acid, they should be eaten with caution by those with kidney stones, or a tendency toward kidney stones. Consult your physician if there is a history of stones in your family.*

BLACK CURRANTS
1 cup, raw

Calories	72
Protein	1.6 gm
Carbohydrate	17.4 gm
Fat	0.6 gm
Cholesterol	0 mg
Dietary Fiber	6.1 gm

	Amount	RDA
Vitamin C	202 mg	337%
Iron	1.8 mg	12%
Vitamin E	1.1 mg	11%
Magnesium	28 mg	7%
Calcium	62 mg	5%
Potassium	360 mg	NA

RED AND WHITE CURRANTS
1 cup, raw

Calories	62
Protein	1.6 gm
Carbohydrate	15.6 gm
Fat	0.4 gm
Cholesterol	0 mg
Dietary Fiber	6.3 gm

	Amount	RDA
Vitamin C	46 mg	77%
Iron	1.2 mg	8%
Potassium	308 mg	NA

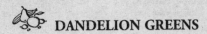 DANDELION GREENS

Although no one is quite sure where this relative of both the sunflower and common lawn weed originated, it has been part of the diet of many cultures for centuries. It has been used to treat liver problems, diarrhea, fevers, skin ailments, and a host of other problems in many countries throughout recorded history. In fact, the scientific name of its genus, *Taraxacum*, is based on the Greek words for disease and cure. Its popular name, dandelion, is a mispronunciation of the French *dent-de-lion*, or "lion's tooth."

Dandelion Greens' Healing Properties

An excellent source of beta-carotene, the "plant form" for vitamin A, dandelion greens help to protect the body against cancer. The relationship between beta-carotene and cervical cancer was studied in 49 women who had precancerous changes in cervical tissues. The women who took in less than average amounts of beta-carotene and vitamin A were 2.75 to 3 times more likely to develop the abnormalities.

In a fascinating study involving the Ifugao tribe of the Philippines, beta-carotene and vitamin A were pitted directly against tobacco, a known carcinogen. The Ifugao chew a tobacco-like mix called betel quid that damages the cells lining the mouth and oral cavity. The amount of damage amongst the oral cavities of the volunteers was measured, and they were given either beta-carotene, vitamin A, a substance called canthaxanthin, or a placebo. Nine weeks later, the amount of cellular damage in the beta-carotene group was cut by over two-thirds, and by half in the vitamin A group.

Dandelion greens also contain small amounts of lecithin and other substances which may prove to be helpful in the treatment of cirrhosis and other liver ailments. The unheralded vegetable also has a diuretic effect, flushing excess fluid out of the body.

Including the Food in Your Diet

Add dandelion greens to your salads often, to strengthen your resistance to cancer. You can also sauté them in just a little bit of oil or margarine.

DANDELION GREENS
1/2 cup chopped, cooked

Calories	17	
Protein	1.0 gm	
Carbohydrate	3.3 gm	
Fat	0.3 gm	
Cholesterol	0 mg	
Dietary Fiber	——	

	Amount	RDA
Vitamin A	608 RE	61%
Vitamin C	9.4 mg	16%
Calcium	73 mg	6%
Iron	0.9 mg	6%
Potassium	121 mg	NA

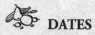 **DATES**

Sweet enough to have been called "candy that comes from trees," dates are roughly 70 percent sugar by weight. Cultivated in the Middle East and North Africa for thousands of years, the carbohydrate-rich fruits sustained caravans traveling across Arabian deserts in ancient times.

The Date's Healing Properties

Good sources of fiber, dates aid the digestive system by speeding matter through the bowels. They also contain potassium and iron, the minerals copper and boron, and a natural aspirin.

Including the Food in Your Diet

An occasional date will sweeten the diet while easing bowel functioning.

DATES		
10 (approx. 3 oz)		
Calories	230	
Protein	1.8 gm	
Carbohydrate	61.3 gm	
Fat	0.4 gm	
Cholesterol	0 mg	
Dietary Fiber	7.0 gm	
	Amount	RDA
Niacin	1.9 mg	10%
Iron	1.0 mg	7%
Folacin	10.4 mcg	5%
Potassium	541 mg	NA

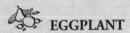 **EGGPLANT**

Native to India or regions nearby, the poor eggplant was viewed with suspicion by most cultures. In fact, the Chinese name for eggplant can be translated as "poison." Northern Europeans steadfastly refused to eat the purple vegetable well into the sixteenth century. The English were sure that anyone who ate eggplant would go insane. In Turkey, Persia, and parts of Africa, however, the eggplant was held in high esteem, being used to treat a variety of ailments, including arthritis, burns, convulsions, and various pains.

The Eggplant's Healing Properties

Low in fat and calories, the eggplant contains terpenes and other substances that show promise as cancer fighters, plus folacin, potassium, and other nutrients. Studies suggest that the eggplant has a mild cholesterol-lowering effect, and may relieve some digestive problems.

Including the Food in Your Diet

Occasionally making eggplant part of five or more daily servings of vegetables and fruits will add variety and taste to your diet. Eggplant can absorb a lot of cooking oil, more so than the average vegetable, so be careful not to use too much oil in preparation. Steaming or boiling the vegetable eliminates this problem.

EGGPLANT ½ cup cubes, cooked		
Calories	13	
Protein	0.4 gm	
Carbohydrate	3.2 gm	
Fat	0.1 gm	
Cholesterol	0 mg	
Dietary Fiber	——	
	Amount	RDA
Folacin	6.9 mcg	3%
Potassium	119 mg	NA

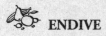 **ENDIVE**

A leafy green vegetable that is sometimes added to salads, and other times cooked like spinach, endive is low in calories and fat. This member of the daisy family is native to India, but spread through the Near East in times of old and was enjoyed by the ancient Egyptians, and later the Greeks and Romans. You probably wouldn't guess by its looks, but endive is related to lettuce and dandelion greens.

Endive's Healing Properties

Endive contains a good amount of folic acid, plus beta-carotene and other nutrients. A member of the B-family of vitamins, folic acid is necessary for growth and the maintenance of a healthy immune system. A lack of folic acid may lead to anemia, anorexia, digestive difficulties, headaches, insomnia, weakness, apathy, and poor memory.

Including the Food in Your Diet

Endive can be steamed, sautéed or otherwise cooked like spinach, or eaten raw in salads. Regularly adding it to your diet a couple of times a week is a simple and tasty way to give your immune system nutrients it can use to fight off disease.

ENDIVE
½ cup chopped, raw

Calories	4	
Protein	0.3 gm	
Carbohydrate	0.8 gm	
Fat	0.1 gm	
Cholesterol	0 mg	
Dietary Fiber	0.5 gm	
	Amount	RDA
Folacin	35.5 mcg	18%
Vitamin A	51 RE	5%

 FIGS

The fig is one of the Western world's oldest and best known medicinal foods. Throughout the ages, the tasty fruit has been used to treat constipation, hemorrhoids, cancer, and other diseases. The Bible tells us that Isaiah cured Hezekiah, an Israeli king who was suffering tremendously from boils, by feeding him figs. During the early days of the United States, Aaron Burr, who later shot Alexander Hamilton, used a spread made from figs to cure his skin infection.

The Fig's Healing Properties

Figs have long been noted for their laxative properties, which are largely due to the high fiber content of the fruit. Figs also contain ficins, enzymes that aid digestion.

The sugary fruit's anticancer properties have been studied by Japanese scientists, who have given cancer patients injections and oral doses of fig extract, resulting in the shrinkage of tumors. Other studies suggest that figs may help to treat ulcers and some parasites.

Including the Food in Your Diet

Adding a few fresh figs a week to your diet will add sweetness to your diet while improving digestion and elimination. Dried figs are, ounce for ounce, higher in nutrients than are fresh figs. (This is because water evaporates from foods when they are dried, leaving the smaller lighter dried food with most of the nutrients of the original "wet" fruit.) Go easy on the dried figs, however, for they are high in sugar.

FIGS, FRESH
1 medium (approx. 1.8 oz)

Calories	37
Protein	0.4 gm
Carbohydrate	9.6 gm
Fat	0.2 gm
Cholesterol	0 mg
Dietary Fiber	1.7 gm

	Amount	RDA
Iron	0.2 mg	13%
Vitamin B_6	.1 mg	5%
Calcium	18 mg	2%
Magnesium	8 mg	2%
Potassium	116 mg	NA

FIGS, DRIED
10 dried (approx. 6.6 oz)

Calories	477
Protein	5.7 gm
Carbohydrate	122.2 gm
Fat	2.2 gm
Cholesterol	0 mg
Dietary Fiber	17 gm

	Amount	RDA
Iron	4.2 mg	28%
Calcium	269 mg	22%
Potassium	1,332 mg	NA

FISH

Anyone born before World War II undoubtedly remembers being forced to swallow a spoonful of cod liver oil on a daily basis—or whenever their mothers thought that they looked a little "sickly." Back then, no one knew exactly why this fish oil improved health, but generations of doctors (and mothers) were convinced that it worked. We finally know why.

Fish's Healing Properties

Fish has been the subject of a great deal of scientific study in the past twenty or so years, especially since Danish researchers began investigating the link between fish-eating Eskimos and their very low rate of heart disease. A great many studies in the medical literature confirm that substances in fish may help to:

- Thin the blood
- Lower blood fat
- Reduce total cholesterol
- Keep blood pressure under control
- Control diabetes
- Relieve headaches
- Reduce the pain and stiffness of arthritis
- Lessen the harmful effects of ulcerative colitis
- Aid in the battle against skin diseases such as eczema and psoriasis

Although more studies are required before definitive statements can be made, early evidence suggests that fish may also be of therapeutic use in treating AIDS, bronchitis, candida, and autoimmune diseases such as lupus.

What Scientists Have Learned About Fish

Fish and the Heart: The link between fish and healthy hearts began to take shape in the early 1970s, when Danish researchers noted that the Eskimos in Greenland suffered from very little coronary heart disease, even though their diets were quite high in fat. In fact, the Eskimo diet consisted largely of fatty fish, whale and seal meat, just the type of diet one would expect to produce a record number of heart attacks.

Much to their surprise, the Danish scientists discovered that something in the fatty fish was acting as a tremendously powerful protector of the heart. This substance apparently thinned the blood, making it less likely to form clots that could lodge in one of the tiny coronary arteries and trigger a heart attack. It also lowered the blood fat, reduced the total cholesterol, and possibly lowered the LDL ("bad") cholesterol.

The mysterious substance turned out to be the "omega-3 fatty acids," which are called "omega-3s" for short. Eating as little as 1 gram of omega-3 fatty acids a day can decrease the risk of coronary artery disease by up to 40 percent. The same omega-3 benefits that protect the heart also reduce the risk of stroke.

Fish and Blood Pressure: Elevated blood pressure (hypertension) is a major contributor to heart disease, stroke, and other potentially deadly diseases. Fortunately, the omega-3s in fish may help to keep the blood pressure at proper levels. A study of 722 men in Finland found that there was an inverse relationship between omega-3s and blood pressure. In other words, the more fish and omega-3s they ate, the lower their blood pressures. Fish oil may also help if the blood pressure is already elevated. Six different studies on patients with mild hypertension found that long-term therapy with fish oil could bring the blood pressure back down to, or close to, normal levels.

Fish and Diabetes: Many diabetics produce enough insulin in their bodies, but they are not as sensitive to their insulin as they should be. Thus, they need extra help from insulin injections. Giving omega-3 fatty acids to these people causes them to become more sensitive to their own insulin. This reduces their dependence on insulin injections, and helps to control the harmful effects of their diabetes. The omega-3s also slow the progressive damage to the blood vessels caused by diabetes, and improve the supply of blood to the heart.

Fish and Headaches: Having noted that the omega-3s seemed to relieve headaches as well, researchers conducted a double-blind study with 15 patients suffering from severe migraine headaches that had not been helped by conventional medications. Eight of the patients reported fewer headaches and less pain upon taking omega-3 supplements. Another study, involving 6 patients suffering from severe, frequent migraines, found that seven ounces of fish oil per day led to a drop in both the frequency and severity of headaches.

Fish and Arthritis: Two 1985 studies reported that giving omega-3s to patients with rheumatoid arthritis resulted in less joint stiffness and tenderness within three months. When the treatment was halted, the patients' joints rapidly became stiffer and more tender.

Omega-3s have also demonstrated their effectiveness against the much more common osteoarthritis. A group of patients ranging in age from 52 to 85 had osteoarthritis pain despite taking ibuprofen daily for two weeks. Some of the patients were given omega-3 oil capsules, while others were given a placebo. The ones who took the fish oil soon had less pain, and were better able to carry on with their usual activities.

Fish and Ulcerative Colitis: Ulcerative colitis is a chronic inflammatory disorder of the large intestine and rectum, producing a watery diarrhea that contains blood, pus, and mucus. Its victims may also suffer from severe abdominal pain, anemia, weight loss, fever and chills, and must often severely restrict their activities. Until recently, strong drugs and surgery were the only available medical treatments for ulcerative colitis.

Hoping to find a milder yet more effective cure for the disease, researchers studied 10 patients suffering from mild to moderate ulcerative colitis. After eight weeks of receiving fish oil, 7 of the 10 reported moderate to marked improvement in their symptoms. Equally encouraging, the doses of prednisone, a medicine with powerful side effects, could be reduced in 4 out of 5 patients who were taking this strong medication.

Fish and Cancer: A number of studies, including the prestigious ''MRFIT'' study, have found an inverse relationship between fish and cancer: The more fish one eats, the less likely he or she is to get cancer, especially of the breast or colon.

Fish and the Skin: Fish oils have shown promise against skin diseases such as eczema and psoriasis. Fish may help to keep the skin healthy because fish oil relieves inflammation, a common symptom of skin diseases. In one study, patients with eczema were given either fish oil or a placebo. After 12 weeks, the ones who received the fish oil reported less itching, scaling, and skin sensitivity.

Fish and Intelligence: Fish has long been considered a "brain food," although no one seemed to know why eating fish might make one smarter. Now some researchers have suggested that the omega-3s may be related to intelligence. When laboratory animals were fed a diet deficient in omega-3 fatty acids, they suffered from impaired learning ability and poor vision.

The Fish With the Most Omega-3 Fatty Acids

Generally speaking, fish that live in cold waters tend to have more omega-3s than do fish from warmer locales. Here is a list of the omega-3 content of some common fish:

Fish (3½ ounces)	Grams of Omega-3s
Norwegian Sardines	5.1
Chinook Salmon	3.0
Atlantic Mackerel	2.2
Pink Salmon	1.9
Sablefish	1.4
Atlantic Herring	1.1
Rainbow Trout	1.1
Pacific Oyster	.8
Striped Bass	.6
Alaskan King Crab	.6
Ocean Perch	.5
Pacific Halibut	.5
Shrimp	.4
Flounder	.3
Haddock	.2

Including the Food in Your Diet

Various studies have shown that eating fish once or twice a week cuts the risk of dying of coronary heart disease by about half. The risk of suffering a stroke is also reduced.

Besides the omega-3s, fish have many other healthy nutrients. Although each fish has a unique "nutrient profile," in general you can count on getting various B-vitamins, magnesium, iron, and potassium by including a variety of fish in your diet.

HERRING
3 oz, baked or broiled

Calories	222	
Protein	19.4 gm	
Carbohydrate	0.4 gm	
Fat	15.4 gm	
Cholesterol	95 mg	
Dietary Fiber	——	

	Amount	RDA
Vitamin B_{12}	0.6 mcg	30%
Vitamin B_6	0.4 mg	20%
Magnesium	34.6 mg	9%
Potassium	475.2 mg	NA

COD
3 oz, baked or broiled

Calories	100	
Protein	17.5 gm	
Carbohydrate	0.3 gm	
Fat	3.2 gm	
Cholesterol	49.6 mg	
Dietary Fiber	——	

	Amount	RDA
Vitamin B_{12}	0.7 mcg	35%
Vitamin B_6	0.2 mg	10%
Phosphorus	118 mg	9%
Magnesium	28.8 mg	7%

HALIBUT
3½ oz, baked or broiled

Calories	140	
Protein	27	gm
Carbohydrate	0	gm
Fat	3	gm
Cholesterol	41	mg
Dietary Fiber	——	

	Amount	RDA
Vitamin B_{12}	1.0 mcg	50%
Niacin	7.0 mg	35%
Magnesium	107 mg	27%
Phosphorus	285 mg	24%
Vitamin B_6	0.4 mg	20%

SALMON
3 oz, baked or broiled

Calories	149
Protein	20.5 gm
Carbohydrate	0.4 gm
Fat	6.8 gm
Cholesterol	35.7 mg
Dietary Fiber	——

	Amount	RDA
Niacin	24.5	122%
Vitamin B_{12}	2.3 mcg	115%
Phosphorus	238 mg	20%

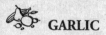 **GARLIC**

Garlic makes a man wink, drink, and stink.
—ENGLISH PROVERB

Although garlic may not drive away vampires, only people, it does have a long history of being used as a medicine and tonic. In ancient times, eating the pungent vegetable was felt to make one strong and courageous. The Chinese credited garlic with curing the cold, tuberculosis, bronchitis, and many other ailments. For Pliny the Elder, a scientist and naturalist who lived during the height of the Roman Empire, garlic was the treatment of choice for more than 60 ailments. Hippocrates, the "Father of Medicine," treated wounds and pneumonia with garlic preparations.

Although physicians, herbalists, and other healers had long trusted garlic's healing properties, it was not until 1858 that Louis Pasteur noted that tiny amounts of garlic could kill bacteria. This was the first scientific proof of garlic's medicinal powers, but almost 90 years passed before allicin, the strong-smelling substance that actually kills bacteria, was extracted from garlic and its medicinal properties recognized.

Garlic's Healing Properties

Garlic contains good amounts of vitamins C and B_6, plus potassium, selenium, phosphorus, quercetin, cyanidin, bioflavonoids, allicin, and more than 70 sulfur compounds (which are responsible for garlic's strong flavor and aroma). Some scientists believe that the jury is still out, while others feel that there is extremely credible scientific evidence that garlic has remarkable healing powers. Studies indicate that garlic may:

- Protect against cancer, especially in the stomach, colon, and rectum
- Help to diminish the signs and symptoms of aging
- Reduce cholesterol
- Protect against heart disease and stroke by "thinning" the blood
- Lower blood pressure

- Relieve arthritis pain
- Have antiviral, antibiotic, and antifungal properties
- Serve as a decongestant, an expectorant to help expel mucus, and an antispasmodic to quiet bronchial spasms associated with asthma and other respiratory problems
- Aid in digestion
- Help to relieve gas
- Help to control diarrhea
- Act as a diuretic to help flush excess water from the body
- Lift the mood and exert a mild calming effect

What Scientists Have Learned About Garlic

Garlic and Cancer: More than 30 substances that help to control cancer have been found in garlic, including ajoene, quercetin, and diallyl sulfide. The diallyl sulfide (DAS) found in garlic oil appears to disarm carcinogens and to slow the rate at which tumors grow.

Studies of large groups of people have shown that those who eat more garlic (and onions) tend to have lower cancer rates. In laboratory and animal studies, garlic or purified substances extracted from garlic have reduced cancers of the breast, colon, and esophagus by up to 75 percent. A study involving over 40,000 women in Iowa found that eating garlic once a week was enough to cut the risk of colon cancer by more than one-third. Due to the wealth of anecdotal and scientific evidence, the National Cancer Institute now supports the idea that garlic is a cancer-slayer.

Garlic and Aging: "Feeding" garlic to cells in test tubes has youth-preserving, anti-aging and beneficial effects on human cells. Scientists believe that garlic may extend life by detoxifying harmful substances that make their way into the body, by protecting cells from the damaging effects of oxidation, by suppressing tumors, and by helping in the battle against bacteria and fungi.

Garlic and Cholesterol: Almost 2,000 years ago, the prominent physician Disocorides noted that garlic helped to keep the arteries open and the blood flowing freely. More recently, researchers have found that adding 1.8 ounces of garlic juice to a high-fat, high-cholesterol meal actually *decreases* the blood cholesterol by some 7 percent. In one long-term study, patients with heart disease and high cholesterol added the equivalent of three cloves of garlic a day to their diets for ten months.

The garlic-eaters enjoyed a significant drop in cholesterol (compared to a control group).

In another study, 62 patients with coronary heart disease and elevated cholesterol levels were divided into two groups. In the group that received garlic for ten months, the cholesterol, blood fat, and bad cholesterol dropped, while the good cholesterol rose.

Garlic and Thin Blood: Although we tend of think of "clogged arteries" as being responsible for heart attacks, many times it only takes a partially blocked artery, plus a blood clot, to trigger the deadly problem. Blood clots continually form and dissolve in the body. If, however, a clot does not dissolve, but instead floats through the bloodstream, it may lodge in a partially narrowed artery in the heart, stopping the flow of blood and triggering a heart attack. The same scenario may be played out in an artery in the brain, causing a stroke.

Fortunately, garlic "thins" the blood. A substance called ajoene in garlic is at least as powerful a blood thinner as is aspirin, which is recommended to patients at risk of heart disease, stroke, or other ailments related to "thick" blood.

Garlic and Blood Pressure: Research on garlic has shown that large amounts of the pungent vegetable (or preparations made from it) can reduce blood pressure. A study of German patients with high blood pressure found that garlic can bring blood pressure down by an average of 20 points within three months, and that the effect gets stronger with time. Garlic's ability to lower blood pressure is at least partially due to the relaxing effect it has on the smooth muscles surrounding blood vessels. As the muscles relax, the vessels expand. In effect, the blood vessels "grow" a little bit wider, thus reducing the pressure.

Garlic and Arthritis: Physicians giving garlic to heart patients who also had arthritis noticed that the garlic seemed to relieve the patients' joint pain. Although garlic's ability to relieve arthritis pain has not been subjected to large-scale tests, it does help the body regulate the mechanisms which bring on inflammation. Furthermore, there are many sulfur-containing compounds in garlic, and it's been known since the 1930s that sulfur supplementation can help arthritis patients.

Garlic and Infection: A powerful, natural, antibacterial agent, garlic destroys or disarms more than 70 different infectious bacteria which cause tuberculosis, encephalitis, diarrhea, botulism, and other serious diseases. Garlic also acts as a broad-spectrum fungal agent that can destroy 17 different strains of fungus.

Including the Food in Your Diet

Although there is no RDA for garlic, nutritionally minded physicians recommend adding garlic to your food whenever possible, up to the equivalent of 3 medium cloves a day. A quick and easy way to add garlic to your diet is to simply chop and mix it in a vegetable stir-fry. Or try roasting a whole head of garlic wrapped in foil in a 350° oven for 45 minutes to 1 hour, then squeeze the garlic on to bread—the taste is surprisingly mild and delicious. Garlic can also be used in dressings; it livens up soups, casseroles, and bread mixes. You can triple the amount of garlic called for in most recipes, which were designed for timid palates.

Eating a little bit of parsley after having garlic will help to freshen the breath. If garlic breath is a problem for you, or those around you, try garlic supplements rather than the real thing. Supplements such as Kyolic™ use aged, odorless garlic that has no unpleasant effect upon the breath. Check the label to see how much should be taken in order to get the equivalent of 3 cloves of garlic a day.

GARLIC
1 oz, raw

Calories	43	
Protein	1.7	gm
Carbohydrate	9	gm
Fat	<1	gm
Saturated Fat	<1	gm
Cholesterol	0	mg
Dietary Fiber	——	

	Amount	RDA
Vitamin B_6	.3 mg	15%
Vitamin C	9 mg	15%

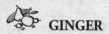 **GINGER**

Ginger has a long history of use as a medicine. Two thousand years ago, the Chinese were using the root to treat fever, diarrhea, coughing, vomiting, and other problems. Ginger has been used as an aphrodisiac in Africa and, at the other end of the spectrum, as a form of birth control in the South Pacific.

Ginger's Healing Properties

Although it is not a nutritionally rich food, ginger has demonstrated medicinal abilities. Studies suggest that ginger may help to:

- Prevent heart attacks by thinning the blood
- Prevent motion sickness

Ginger is also reported to be helpful in relieving arthritis, migraine headaches, heartburn, and gas. Laboratory studies have shown that it has antiviral and antibacterial properties as well, and may help to "rev up" the metabolism and burn off calories.

What Scientists Have Learned About Ginger

Ginger and the Blood: Like garlic and onions, ginger helps to thin the blood and prevent unwanted, possibly dangerous blood clots that can trigger heart attacks and strokes. A complicated series of events is necessary before blood can clot. Ginger's ability to interfere with the series was accidentally discovered by a doctor at Cornell University who, while conducting a routine analysis of his own blood, noticed that it was not coagulating as rapidly as it normally did. Remembering that he had eaten some ginger the night before, he fed ginger to his fellow researchers and then checked their blood. His studies showed that ginger definitely "thinned" the blood, and could help to prevent unwanted, possibly dangerous blood clots.

Ginger, Motion Sickness, and Nausea: The Chinese have long used ginger to prevent or ameliorate seasickness. In a test that might even give NASA astronauts trouble, volunteers were strapped into a special chair and spun about, tilted back and forth, and generally tossed about. The volunteers who had been previously given powdered ginger root lasted much longer in the chair than did those given either Dramamine™ or a placebo.

Intrigued by the reports that ginger helps to settle upset stomachs, anesthesiologists have looked into ginger's ability to prevent or reduce the nausea and vomiting that so often accompanies general anesthesia. Ginger's antinausea abilities were studied in a double-blind study in which one group of women was given an antinausea drug, while a second group took ginger capsules. The ginger group fared better than those who were given the medicine. Ginger is also helpful for pregnant women suffering from nausea.

Including the Food in Your Diet

About ½ teaspoon of ginger is usually enough to prevent or reduce motion sickness in most people. Add plenty of ginger to your diet by chopping it up and adding it to vegetable stir-frys and rice dishes. It also can be used in curries and baked dishes, and even in fruit salads.

GINGER
1 Tablespoon

Calories	4	
Protein	0.1 gm	
Carbohydrate	0.9 gm	
Fat	0.1 gm	
Cholesterol	0 mg	
Dietary Fiber	0.1 gm	
	Amount	RDA
Potassium	46 mg	NA

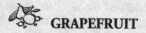

GRAPEFRUIT

Writing some 300 years before the birth of Christ, a Greek scholar noted that grapefruit pulp sweetened the breath and was an antidote to poison.

Food historians feel that grapefruit is the child of a "marriage" between the orange and a sour, dry citrus fruit called the shaddock. Through the years, careful breeding has improved the flavor and texture of the grapefruit. Unfortunately for dieters, eating grapefruit does not magically cause the pounds to melt away. However, this citrus fruit is good for the heart, has little fat or salt, and contains excellent amounts of vitamin C, as well as folic acid, fiber, and potassium.

The Grapefruit's Healing Properties

Although its healing powers are not as well known as those of the orange or garlic, grapefruit packs a medicinal wallop. Studies have shown that it may:

- Lower cholesterol
- Help the body eliminate older ineffective red blood cells
- Reduce the risk of pancreatic and other cancers
- Strengthen the immune system and improve general health

What Scientists Have Learned About the Grapefruit

Grapefruit and Cholesterol: Grapefruit pulp contains soluble fibers, such as pectin, that may go beyond simply lowering the total cholesterol: Grapefruit also lowers the LDL ("bad") cholesterol and may "clean out" clogged arteries by stripping away the dangerous plaque/fat/debris deposits.

Grapefruit's ability to lower cholesterol was put to the test at the University of Florida when 27 adults were given either a "grapefruit pill" containing grapefruit pectin, or a placebo, three times per day. (They weren't told if they were getting the real thing or the placebo until the study was over.) Within 8 weeks, total cholesterol levels in the ones who had taken the "grapefruit pills" fell by 7.6 percent, while their LDL ("bad") cholesterol dropped almost 11 percent.

Grapefruit and Red Blood Cells: Human blood contains a complex mix of substances, including fluid, red blood cells, white blood cells, and platelets. The red blood cells ferry oxygen from the lungs, through the bloodstream and to every part of the body. There should be enough red blood cells to transport the oxygen, but not so many that they make the blood sludgy and thick, increasing the risk of heart disease. (Too few red blood cells to carry oxygen, on the other hand, is associated with anemia.)

Doctors monitor the red blood cells by measuring the hematocrit, the percent of red blood cells in the blood. For men, a normal hematocrit ranges from 40 to 55 percent, while for women the range is 37 to 47 percent.

Recent studies have found that a flavonoid in grapefruit called naringin helps to lower elevated hematocrits by encouraging the body to "chew up" and destroy older red blood cells that are no longer efficient, but remain in the blood and make it "thick." (Surprisingly, naringin also appears to raise low hematocrit levels, although how it does so is not well understood.)

Grapefruit and Cancer: Citrus fruits, including grapefruit, contain some 50-plus substances that fight against cancer, including antioxidants, carotenoids, coumarins, flavonoids, limonoids, and terpenes. And the "bundling" of these cancer-fighters in these fruits makes them stronger than they would be individually.

Researchers have long known that those living in countries or regions where large amounts of citrus fruits are eaten tend to get less cancer than do those living in areas where citrus fruit is a less common part of the diet. This citrus fruit–cancer connection has been confirmed by many researchers in various countries.

Swedish researchers have compared people who regularly ate citrus fruit (one a day) to those who rarely consumed citrus (one a week). The one-a-dayers had less than half the risk of suffering from pancreatic cancer. Japanese scientists have tested grapefruit's anticancer abilities by injecting it into special mice, where it stopped tumors from growing and brought about complete or partial remission from cancer.

Ruby red grapefruit contains a cancer-fighting carotenoid called lycopene. Various studies have found that low levels of lycopene in the blood are associated with greater risks of cancer of the cervix, bladder, and pancreas. And, of course, the lycopene and other antioxidants in grapefruit help the body control the potentially cancer-causing damage of oxidation.

Grapefruit, the Immune System, and General Health: A single grapefruit, or 8 ounces of fresh grapefruit juice, contain more than 100 percent of the RDA for vitamin C. One of C's most important duties is strengthening the immune system by stimulating T-cells, B-cells, and the "cell eaters" (macrophages) that ingest and destroy bacteria, viruses, and other invaders. The vitamin helps to protect the heart by regulating the liver's production of cholesterol and by helping to remove cholesterol from artery walls. It also helps asthmatics breathe easier, and can speed up recovery from pneumonia, mononucleosis, hepatitis, and other viral infections.

Including the Food in Your Diet

Eating a single grapefruit every day can significantly lower your risk of pancreatic cancer. Beginning each day with half a grapefruit at breakfast, followed by more citrus or other fruit later in the day, is a delicious way to increase your resistance to cancer, heart disease, and many other avoidable ailments.

Grapefruit's pectin is found in the pulpy sections, so be sure to eat the pulpy membrane that separates the individual sections.

Caution: The naringin and other flavonoids in grapefruit may interfere with the body's ability to properly metabolize certain medications, including calcium channel blockers such as Procardia (nifedipine) and Plendil (felodipine), and antihistamines such as Seldane D. If you are taking these or any other prescription or over-the-counter medications, ask your physician about possible interactions or other problems that may occur if you eat grapefruit or drink grapefruit juice.

GRAPEFRUIT
½ raw (approx. 4 oz)

Calories	39
Protein	0.8 gm
Carbohydrate	9.9 gm
Fat	0.1 gm
Cholesterol	0 mg
Dietary Fiber	0.7 gm

	Amount	RDA
Vitamin C	39.3 mg	66%
Folacin	11.8 mcg	6%

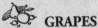 **GRAPES**

Cultivated perhaps as long as 5,000 years ago, grapes were the "fruit of the vine" referred to in the Bible. Grapes are commonly classified as "European" or "American." European varieties include Thompson Seedless, Flame Seedless, and Red Globe grapes. American varieties, with skin that usually slips easily off the flesh, include Concord, Steuben, and Delaware grapes.

The Grape's Healing Properties

Although grapes contain well-known nutrients such as vitamin C, thiamin, vitamin B_6, potassium, and riboflavin, other lesser-known substances such as ellagic acid and resveratrol in the small fruit give surprising health benefits. Grapes may help to:

• Fight cancer
• Increase good cholesterol
• Thin the blood

Red grapes are very good sources of the mineral selenium, and contain the bone-building mineral boron.

What Scientists Have Learned About the Grape

Grapes and Cancer: Grapes, certain nuts, and strawberries have large concentrations of ellagic acid, a powerful inhibitor of mutagenesis, as well as caffeic acid, which has proven its ability to fight cancers in animals. In a study with laboratory mice, an extract taken from Concord grapes slowed tumor growth as effectively as did methotrexate, a cancer drug. Red grapes also contain quercetin, an antioxidant that helps to fight cancer, protect the heart, and slow the effects of aging.

Unfortunately, researchers have not yet turned much of their attention to grapes. Thus, the fruit's promising anticancer potential has not been fully explored thus far.

Grapes and the Heart: A substance in grape skin called resveratrol protects against heart disease by increasing HDL cholesterol. Resveratrol also helps to prevent unnecessary blood clots from forming inside the body. This, in turn, helps to keep the blood flowing and to cut back on heart attacks, strokes, and other potentially serious problems.

Grapeseed oil has also been found to raise the HDL. In tests at the State University of New York Health Science Center, half of the women on a low-fat diet plus grapeseed oil saw their HDLs rise by an average of 14 percent.

Including the Food in Your Diet

When they're in season, add grapes to your fruit salads, or eat them by themselves as a snack a couple of times a week. They're also surprisingly delicious when cut in half and added to fish dishes.

GRAPES
European types such as Thompson
1 cup, raw

Calories	114
Protein	1.1 gm
Carbohydrate	28.4 gm
Fat	0.9 gm
Cholesterol	0 mg
Dietary Fiber	1.1 gm

	Amount	RDA
Vitamin C	17.3 mg	29%
Thiamin	0.2 mg	13%
Vitamin B$_6$	0.2 mg	10%
Riboflavin	0.1 mg	6%
Potassium	296 mg	NA

GRAPES
American types such as Concord
1 cup, raw

Calories	60
Protein	0.6 gm
Carbohydrate	16 gm
Fat	0.4 gm
Cholesterol	0 mg
Dietary Fiber	0.6 gm

	Amount	RDA
Vitamin C	4 mg	6%
Potassium	176 mg	NA

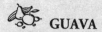 **GUAVA**

Native to the Caribbean, the guava comes in many varieties. Different varieties of the fruit vary in thickness from 1 to 5 inches in circumference, and may be round like an apple or more pear-shaped. Depending on the variety chosen, and the freshness, the taste can range from sweet to sour. There may also be mild taste "hints" of other fruits, such as strawberry or banana.

The Guava's Healing Properties

The guava is low in fat and calories but high in vitamin C and fiber such as pectin. It also contains beta-carotene and potassium. The guava may help to:

* Strengthen the immune system
* Lower cholesterol
* Reduce the risk of colon cancer

What Scientists Have Learned About the Guava

Guava, Vitamin C, and the Immune System: The guava is a superlative source of vitamin C, with a single fruit containing more than 250 percent of the RDA for that powerful nutrient. Vitamin C strengthens the immune system, increasing the mobility of the white blood cells that engage viruses, bacteria, and other invaders in hand-to-hand combat. It has been used to speed up the recovery from hepatitis, pneumonia, mononucleosis, and other viral infections. Vitamin C, which acts as an antihistamine, may reduce the symptoms of seasonal allergic rhinitis (allergies that plague the nose). In its antioxidant capacity, C helps to protect the heart and the rest of the body from the ravages of oxidation. It can also slow the onset of the signs and symptoms of aging.

Guava and Pectin: In addition to vitamin C, guava contains pectin, a fiber that helps to lower both total cholesterol and LDL ("bad") cholesterol. Pectin also helps to reduce the harmful side effects of diabetes by keeping the blood sugar under control.

The pectin in guava also helps to reduce the risk of colon cancer. Researchers at the University of Texas Health Sciences Center have found that feeding pectin to laboratory animals lowers the rate of colon cancer by up to 50 percent. The enormous amounts of vitamin C, plus the small supply of beta-carotene in guava, also help to control cancer.

Including the Food in Your Diet

Making guava a regular part of your fruit intake, when guava is in season, will help to keep your immune system strong and reduce the risk of cancer.

GUAVA 1 raw (approx. 2.7 oz)		
Calories	46	
Protein	0.8 gm	
Carbohydrate	11.4 gm	
Fat	0.4 gm	
Cholesterol	0 mg	
Dietary Fiber	4.5 gm	
	Amount	RDA
Vitamin C	165.1 mg	275%
Vitamin B$_6$	0.2 mg	10%
Vitamin A	71 RE	7%
Niacin	1.1 mg	6%
Potassium	25.6 mg	NA

 KALE

Best known as a leaf to decorate dishes and as a food for livestock, kale has never been a culinary favorite. That's a shame, for kale is a member of the cancer-fighting crucifer family of vegetables.

Kale's Healing Properties

Kale is practically fat-free, has very good amounts of vitamin C and beta-carotene, and also supplies iron, magnesium, calcium, and fiber.

Very closely related to collards, kale contains beta-carotene, vitamin C, lutein, chlorophyll, indoles, sulforaphane, and other powerful cancer-fighters that help to reduce the risk of cancer of the bladder, lung, prostate, bowel, and other parts of the body. These and other substances in kale may also help lower blood pressure, while protecting against heart disease and stroke.

Just ½ cup of kale contains over 40 percent of the RDA for vitamin C and beta-carotene, two nutrients that strengthen the immune system, reduce the risk of heart disease and stroke, and may even delay the onset of the signs and symptoms of aging.

Including the Food in Your Diet

A cancer-fighting crucifer, kale should be a regular part of the diet. It can be quickly and easily chopped up and added to salads, or to many recipes calling for spinach, lettuce, or other greens. It's delicious added to stir-fries with lots of garlic, or as an addition to pasta sauces.

KALE
½ cup chopped, cooked

Calories	21	
Protein	1.2 gm	
Carbohydrate	3.7 gm	
Fat	0.3 gm	
Cholesterol	0 mg	
Dietary Fiber	———	

	Amount	RDA
Vitamin A	481 RE	48%
Vitamin C	26.7 mg	45%
Iron	0.6 mg	4%

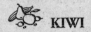 **KIWI**

Although named after New Zealand's kiwi bird, the kiwi is actually from China, where it has been traditionally used to treat some forms of cancer.

The Kiwi's Healing Properties

Rich in vitamin C, the kiwi also provides fiber, potassium, beta-carotene, and niacin. It has little fat or sodium.

A single large kiwi provides more than 100 percent of the RDA for vitamin C. This means that eating kiwi helps to bolster the body's ability to fight cancer, to reduce the risk of heart disease, to guard against oxidation damage to body cells, and to keep a man's sperm lively and healthy.

In addition, the 4.5 grams of dietary fiber found in a single kiwi help to regulate blood sugar. The fiber also offers protection against constipation and hemorrhoids, as well as cancers of the colon, rectum, pancreas, prostate, and breast.

Including the Food in Your Diet

Eating several kiwi per week, when they are in season, will help to keep your immune system strong.

```
                        KIWI
            1 raw (approx. 2.7 oz)

    Calories        46
    Protein            0.8 gm
    Carbohydrate      11.4 gm
    Fat                0.4 gm
    Cholesterol     ——
    Dietary Fiber      4.5 gm

                    Amount          RDA
    Vitamin C       74.5            124%
    Niacin           0.4 mg           2%
    Vitamin A       13   RE           1%
    Potassium      252   mg          NA
```

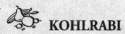

KOHLRABI

A blend of cabbage and turnip, kohlrabi has a rather embarrassing history. Charlemagne the Great, founder of the Holy Roman Empire, ordered that kohlrabi be planted in his domain but only be fed to cattle. (It seems that his doctor had warned him that eating kohlrabi would make one "cow-ish.") Early Americans had equally scant regard for the vegetable. Seed catalogs of the nineteenth century noted that if the kids refused to eat the kohlrabi, it could always be fed to the cattle.

Kohlrabi is a crucifer, a cancer-fighting member of the family that includes cauliflower, Brussels sprouts, cabbage, kale, broccoli, mustard greens, watercress, and radishes.

Kohlrabi's Healing Properties

An excellent source of vitamin C, kohlrabi also contains vitamin E, potassium, and B_6. The vitamin C in kohlrabi may help to strengthen the immune system, speed up recovery from infectious diseases, assist in the removal of dangerous cholesterol from artery walls, check rampaging oxidants, guard against cancer, and make breathing easier for asthmatics.

Kohlrabi contains indoles, phenols, coumarins, and other substances that lower the odds of suffering from various cancers, including cancer of the bladder, lung, prostate, and bowel. The incidence of fibrocystic breast disease—those small, noncancerous, sometimes painful lumps in the breast—can also be reduced by eating cruciferous vegetables.

Including the Food in Your Diet

Like the other crucifers, kohlrabi is an excellent cancer-fighter that should be eaten regularly. Most people prefer to eat it chopped up, in salads. It's also easy to add to soups and stews.

KOHLRABI
½ cup slices, cooked

Calories	24	
Protein	1.5 gm	
Carbohydrate	5.5 gm	
Fat	0.1 gm	
Cholesterol	0 mg	
Dietary Fiber	0.9 gm	

	Amount	RDA
Vitamin C	44 mg	73%
Vitamin B$_6$	0.1 mg	5%
Potassium	279 mg	NA

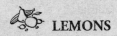 **LEMONS**

Is lemon juice a cure for snakebite? The ancient Romans believed that if you were lucky enough to have eaten a lemon before being bitten by a poisonous snake, you would survive. In other cultures, the lemon was used to treat sore throats, wounds, skin problems, and "bloating."

The Lemon's Healing Properties

Experiments with lemons, conducted some two hundred years ago on grateful sailors of the British and Dutch navies, are perhaps the oldest nutrition studies. Like explorers, soldiers and others who had to go without eating fresh fruits and vegetables for long periods of time, the sailors were often afflicted with scurvy, an eventually fatal disease. Fortunately, the British and Dutch navies found that feeding their sailors fresh lemons or limes, or the juice of the fruits, cured the problem, although they were not sure why. Today we know that it was the vitamin C in the lemons and limes that cured the seafarers. The former scourge is no longer a major problem, for a single lemon contains half the RDA for C, and less than two tablespoons of lemon juice a day will provide enough of the vitamin to prevent scurvy.

The lemon's vitamin C also strengthens the immune system, and speeds the healing of wounds. Terpenes, limonene, glucarase, and flavonoids in lemons help to prevent or slow the growth of certain cancers. Some of the flavonoids found in lemons are also antioxidants that work with vitamin C to guard against heart disease, the ravages of aging, and other problems.

Including the Food in Your Diet

Consuming more than two tablespoons a day will help to strengthen the immune system and bolster your resistance to many diseases. Use generous amounts of lemon juice as a seasoning on vegetables, fruit salads, and fish, and drink fresh lemonade often.

LEMON JUICE
1 tablespoon

Calories	4
Protein	0.1 gm
Carbohydrate	1.4 gm
Fat	0 gm
Cholesterol	0 mg
Dietary Fiber	0 gm

	Amount	RDA
Vitamin C	75% mg	11%

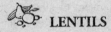 LENTILS

Lentils have an ancient, but unfortunately tainted, history. It was, after all, for a bowl of lentils that Esau sold his birthright to brother Jacob in the Bible.

Lentils are legumes, which means that they are closely related to peas and beans (including the carob bean). The small, round lentils come in three colors: brown, green, and red.

Lentils' Healing Properties

Just ½ cup of cooked lentils contains 86 percent of the RDA for folic acid, a vitamin which plays a dual role in fighting cancer. On one hand, it helps to prevent cancer-causing mutations to body cells by regulating cell division and by maintaining healthy DNA and RNA. And, thanks to its ability to strengthen the immune system, folic acid helps the body fight cancers that do arise.

Lentils contain a small amount of copper, a mineral which helps to control cancer, keep the bones strong, and possibly regulate pain perception. The 2.7 grams of soluble and insoluble fibers in ½ cup of cooked lentils helps to protect against cancers of the colon, rectum, pancreas, prostate, and breast.

By making the stool soft and bulky, fiber speeds its transit through the bowls, reducing constipation, straining upon elimination, and hemorrhoids. The fiber in lentils also helps diabetics keep their blood sugar under control, reducing the risk of diabetic damage to the blood vessels, heart, eyes, and other parts of the body.

Lentils are high in protein but low in fat and calories. They contain phytates, which help body cells to resist cancerous changes, as well as iron, potassium, magnesium, and zinc.

Including the Food in Your Diet

Lentils can be cooked and eaten like beans, made into soup, mixed with rice, or added to many recipes. Sprouted lentils, which look like little round brown or red discs, are delicious additions to salads and sandwiches. By themselves, in soups, in salads, or otherwise, lentils should be eaten several times a week.

LENTILS
½ cup, cooked

Calories	101	
Protein	7.4 gm	
Carbohydrate	18.4 gm	
Fat	0 gm	
Cholesterol	0 mg	
Dietary Fiber	2.7 gm	

	Amount	RDA
Folacin	172.7 mcg	86%
Iron	2.3 mg	15%
Thiamin	0.1 mg	7%

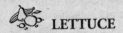 **LETTUCE**

Although the modern American eats approximately 30 pounds of lettuce a year, back in Elizabethan times the vegetable was viewed with suspicion. The merry olde English felt that if married people ate too much lettuce they would become less fertile, and the children they did have would be foolish and resentful.

Other cultures have taken a more charitable view toward this member of the daisy family. The Romans used lettuce as a mild sedative. Lettuce teas and juices had a similar use during colonial times in America, and lettuce extracts continued to be used as a sedative right up until World War II.

Although over eighty varieties of lettuce were known in the United States in the late 1800s, today many supermarkets carry only four basic types: butterhead, looseleaf, Romaine, and iceberg.

Lettuce's Healing Properties

As do many green, leafy vegetables, lettuce contains beta-carotene, folic acid, vitamin K, chlorophyll, lutein, and other substances which strengthen the immune system and improve overall health. Chlorophyll, a natural pigment which gives vegetables their green color, has powerful anticancer and antioxidant properties. In supplement form, chlorophyll is used to treat skin and stomach ulcers, as well as body odor.

The darker and greener the lettuce, the greater the concentration of chlorophyll and other important ingredients. (Iceberg lettuce is the least nutritious of all the lettuces.)

Including the Food in Your Diet

Eat some lettuce with every meal, or have a salad. Be careful not to drown the lettuce in high-fat dressing. Instead, use lemon juice or other fruit juice as a topping.

LETTUCE, ROMAINE
½ cup shredded, raw

Calories	5
Protein	0.5 gm
Carbohydrate	0.7 gm
Fat	< 0.1 gm
Cholesterol	0 mg
Dietary Fiber	0.5 gm

	Amount	RDA
Folacin	38 mcg	19%
Vitamin C	7 mg	12%
Vitamin A	73 RE	7%
Iron	0.3 mg	2%

LETTUCE, RED LEAF
½ cup shredded, raw

Calories	5
Protein	.35 gm
Carbohydrate	1.0 gm
Fat	0.1 gm
Cholesterol	0 mg
Dietary Fiber	0.5 gm

	Amount	RDA
Vitamin C	5 mg	8%
Folacin	14 mcg	7%
Vitamin A	53 RE	5%
Iron	0.4 mg	3%

LETTUCE, ICEBERG
½ cup shredded, raw

Calories	9	
Protein	0.7 gm	
Carbohydrate	1.4 gm	
Fat	0.15 gm	
Cholesterol	0 mg	
Dietary Fiber	——	

	Amount	RDA
Folacin	38 mcg	19%
Vitamin C	2.5 mg	4%

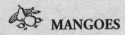 MANGOES

Native to Southeast Asia or India, the mango is mentioned in Hindu mythology, and was praised in a fourteenth-century poem as "the choicest fruit in Hindustan." Mangoes come in hundreds of varieties, sizes, and shapes.

The Mango's Healing Properties

The average-size mango contains approximately 90 percent of the RDA for vitamin C, 75 percent of the RDA for beta-carotene, plus vitamin E and fiber. Together these four substances help to prevent cancers of the colon, rectum, pancreas, prostate, breast, cervix, stomach, and other parts of the body. Beta-carotene and vitamins C and E fight cancer in two ways. First, as antioxidants, they help control the oxidative changes that can turn normal cells cancerous. Second, the vitamins strengthen the immune system, the body's "Department of Defense," which wages war on cancer.

Vitamin C's prowess against cancer is well established. It may also help strengthen the effects of radiation treatment in people who already have cancer. In one study, doctors gave one group of cancer patients radiation therapy, while another group received radiation therapy plus 5 grams (.18 oz) of vitamin C a day. Four months later, the disease had disappeared in 63 percent of those who received C, compared to only 45 percent of those who did not get the vitamin.

An interesting study showed how vitamin E also works against cancer. A group of 766 people with cancer and 1,149 matched controls had their blood drawn *before* cancer was diagnosed. After the doctors knew who had cancer and who did not, they went back and measured the levels of vitamin E in the blood serum (fluid). The people with low levels of a form of vitamin E called alpha-tocopherol were *1½ times more likely to get cancer* than those with higher levels.

Including the Food in Your Diet

A excellent source of immune system–boosting vitamin C and beta-carotene, mangoes should be eaten several times a week when in season. They're delicious plain, or mixed in a fruit salad.

MANGOES
1 raw (approx. 7 oz)

Calories	128	
Protein	1.0	gm
Carbohydrate	33.4	gm
Fat	0.57	gm
Cholesterol	0	mg
Dietary Fiber	2.2	gm

	Amount		RDA
Vitamin C	54	mg	90%
Vitamin A	766	RE	77%
Vitamin E	2.4	mg	24%
Vitamin B_6	.28	mg	14%

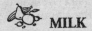 **MILK**

No one knows when the first human drank milk from a cow, goat, or other animal, but it might be as early as 10,000 B.C., when goats were domesticated. Cows were domesticated by 8500 B.C., so we humans have may have been drinking milk from animals for 10,000 to 12,000 years.

That milk was common in the Middle East of biblical times is suggested by many references to the fluid in early writings such as the Bible. The Hebrews are told that the Promised Land is "flowing with milk," and Job laments that God has harmed him and "poured me out as milk."

The ancient Greeks of the fifth century B.C. liked cheese, but felt that drinking milk was beneath them—that was for the barbarians, whom they contemptuously referred to as "milk drinkers." The Romans, who conquered the Greeks, felt the same way about drinking milk. Upper-class Roman ladies, however, valued it highly: for soaking, not for drinking. Bathing in milk was supposed to make the skin soft and white.

Although sometimes criticized as a "kiddie food" or for being "mucus forming," milk really does have something for everybody: calcium, vitamin B_{12}, phosphorus, riboflavin, vitamin D, and the natural amino acid tryptophan.

Milk's Healing Properties

Thanks to its calcium, tryptophan, and other nutrients, milk helps to:

- Keep bones strong
- Prevent high blood pressure
- Relieve insomnia

What Scientists Have Learned About Milk

Milk and Strong Bones: Together calcium, phosphorus, and vitamin D are a powerful trio of bone-builders. Calcium's primary function is to aid in the development and maintenance of bones and teeth. Since bones are continually being reformed throughout life, good supplies of calcium are necessary even into old age. The phosphorus in milk is also vital for healthy bones and teeth. Phosphorus is the second most abundant mineral in the human body, and 80 percent of the body's phosphorus is bound up in the bones and teeth.

Along with calcium and phosphorus, the vitamin D that is added to milk helps to solidify bones and teeth. Before vitamin D was added to milk early in this century, a bone disease called rickets was a major problem (see Chapter Two).

Milk and Blood Pressure: Although we commonly think of excess salt as the cause of high blood pressure, the First National Health & Nutrition Examination Survey found that low-calcium, not high-sodium levels, may be most directly related to high blood pressure. Specifically, the study found that people with high blood pressure consumed 18 percent less calcium than did people with normal levels. A similar study of over 7,000 men of Japanese descent came to a similar conclusion: higher levels of calcium and potassium offered protection against elevated blood pressure.

Although exact figures are hard to determine, it is believed that 700 to 800 milligrams of calcium (about 2 glasses of milk) per day may be enough to ensure that high blood pressure will not develop from a lack of calcium. (There are other causes of elevated blood pressure, however, including hardening of the arteries, chronic kidney disease, and endocrine disorders.)

Milk and Insomnia: People suffering from insomnia, the most common sleep disorder, have difficulty falling asleep or staying asleep, and often find themselves waking up too early in the morning. Many ailments can cause insomnia, including anxiety, depression, chronic pain, and even certain medications, including decongestants and cortisone drugs. Deficiencies of vitamin B_6 or niacin may also be to blame.

Many cases of insomnia are helped by eating foods rich in tryptophan before going to sleep. The body converts tryptophan into serotonin, a neurotransmitter that plays a major role in inducing sleep. Milk, which contains good amounts of tryptophan, has been used as a gentle sleep-inducer for many years.

Milk, Healthy Muscles, and "Good" Nerves: Besides helping to keep blood pressure at the proper levels and the bones strong, milk's calcium is necessary for healthy muscles and nerves. Calcium helps to prevent muscle cramps, irregular heartbeat, and skin problems, plus certain types of depression, delusions and cognitive impairment. Along with vitamin D, calcium is believed to help protect against colon cancer.

The vitamin B_{12} has shown value in treating psoriasis, a common skin disorder that can leave large areas of skin covered with red patches and thick, dry scales.

Including the Drink in Your Diet

Drinking low-fat or nonfat milk every day helps young bones to grow, and provides calcium to keep older bones in shape. Menopausal women should be especially careful to make sure they take in enough calcium (1500 mg per day). Premenopausal women need approximately 1000 mg of calcium a day. To make sure they get this, it is suggested that they drink either two glasses of skim milk and eat one cup of yogurt per day, or have two cups of yogurt and one glass of milk.

Regular (whole) milk is high in fat, and contains cholesterol. Low-fat or nonfat milk is a nutritious alternative that provides the benefits of milk without the excess fat.

Adults also may develop lactose intolerance, an inability to digest the lactose molecules in milk, which results in gastrointestinal distress. Lactose-intolerant adults are often able to drink acidophilus milk, or milk in which the lactose has already been split (Lactaid®). Pills that help one digest lactose are also available. Those who cannot drink milk because of allergies or lactose intolerance may look to tofu, cheeses, or yogurt for their calcium.

```
                    MILK, SKIM
                      1 cup

    Calories            90
    Protein             8.7 gm
    Carbohydrate        12.3 gm
    Fat                 0.6 gm
    Cholesterol         4.9 mg
    Fiber               0   gm

                        Amount          RDA
    Vitamin B₁₂         0.9 mcg         45%
    Calcium             316.3 mg        26%
    Riboflavin          0.4 mg          22%
    Folacin             13.2 mcg         7%
    Potassium           418.2 mg        NA
```

 MUSHROOMS

Mushrooms have long been enjoyed for their delicious flavor and texture. In fact, ancient Egyptian pharaohs considered mushrooms to be a food fit for royalty. Mushrooms have also enjoyed favor in the Orient as a medicine. The Chinese have long felt that mushrooms enhance and extend the lifespan, and use mushrooms to treat viral and other diseases.

The Mushroom's Healing Properties

The fat-free, low-calorie mushroom is a good source of riboflavin and niacin. Mushrooms may:

- Thin the blood
- Lower cholesterol
- Have anticancer properties
- Strengthen the immune system

What Scientists Have Learned About the Mushroom

Mushrooms and the Blood: Until recently, not much was known about the health value of mushrooms in the United States, primarily because the "button" mushroom favored here is not a medicinal standout. Fortunately, Dr. Dale Hammerschmidt of the University of Minnesota enjoyed adding tree ear mushrooms to the Chinese foods he prepared. By chance, while using his own blood in an experiment, he discovered that something in the tree ear mushrooms prevented his platelets from clumping together and causing blood clots. (This is good, for unwanted blood clots and "thick blood" are major contributors to heart disease.)

When Dr. Hammerschmidt published his mushroom/blood findings in the *New England Journal of Medicine,* his report was seen by the researchers who had identified adenosine, an anti-platelet-clumping factor found in garlic and onions. These scientists quickly found that the tree ear mushroom also contained adenosine, plus other blood thinners.

Mushrooms and Cholesterol: Shiitake mushrooms have been found to lower cholesterol by 10 percent or more. In one study, even when butter was added to the diet of volunteers, eating three ounces of shiitake mushrooms a day pushed cholesterol down by 4 percent.

Mushrooms, Cancer, and the Immune System: Substances in shiitake mushrooms rev up the immune system by strengthening the T-cells and the giant macrophages, and by encouraging the production of additional interferon. Interferon is a potent immune-system soldier which aids the immune system in the battle against viruses and cancer.

Eating mushrooms also increases the manufacture of interleukin-1 and interleukin-2. These two immune-system substances help the body to fight tumors and other problems. The tree ear, enoki, and oyster mushrooms have also been found to have anticancer properties in animal studies.

Including the Food in Your Diet

Making mushrooms a regular part of your daily intake of five or more servings of vegetables and fruits will help to prevent heart disease and cancer, while strengthening the immune system.

Which mushrooms you eat can make a difference to your health. As stated, the common "button" mushroom popular in the U.S. is not known to have the powerful medicinal effects possessed by the Asian mushrooms, particularly the shiitake and tree ear mushroom.

Shiitake mushrooms are also known as Chinese black mushrooms, black forest mushrooms, Oriental black mushrooms, and golden oak mushrooms. Wood ear mushrooms are also called tree ear mushrooms and black tree fungus.

Many varieties of mushroom are poisonous, so it's best to get your mushrooms from the market, not from the backyard or a nearby wooded area.

"BUTTON" MUSHROOM
½ cup pieces, cooked

Calories	21	
Protein	1.7 gm	
Carbohydrate	4.0 gm	
Fat	0.4 gm	
Cholesterol	0 mg	
Dietary Fiber	1.7 gm	

	Amount	RDA
Niacin	3.5 mg	18%
Riboflavin	0.2 mg	11%
Iron	1.0 mg	7%
Folacin	14.4 mcg	7%
Potassium	278 mg	NA

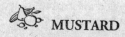 **MUSTARD**

The ancient Chinese considered mustard seeds to be an aid to those who were having sexual difficulties. During the Middle Ages, mustard was used to treat coughs and asthma, and to check congestion and other respiratory problems. Mustard plasters for chest conditions were popular well into the twentieth century. (My father still shudders as he describes the mustard plasters his mother slapped on his chest every time he coughed "suspiciously.")

Mustard's Healing Properties

Although medical science has not yet turned its investigatory eye toward mustard, many researchers feel that it may reduce the severity of respiratory diseases. Like chili and other hot foods, mustard may help to clear the airways of excess mucus. Normally, tiny hairlike projections called cilia move the mucus through the respiratory system and up toward the throat. If the cilia are damaged by disease, or if the mucus becomes too thick and sticky, it may remain in the airways, interfering with breathing. Mustard and other hot foods may help to clear the mucus from the airways, possibly by irritating certain nerves that trigger the release of fluids which wash the mucus away.

Mustard also contains magnesium, which helps to prevent cancer and heart disease. Dieters, take note: Mustard may help you burn off more calories by speeding up the metabolism.

As for those mustard plasters, it seems that mustard (and horseradish) contains allylisothiocyanate, an oil which can relieve pain by causing irritation and increasing blood flow when applied to the skin. Be careful, however, for applying mustard directly on the skin can cause blistering. Check with your physician before using a mustard plaster.

Including the Food in Your Diet

Mustard is made up of dry mustard powder, vinegar, water, and spices. Prepared mustards, whether yellow or brown, tend to be high in sodium. Many of us already add mustard to meat or fish dishes. Try dabbing a little on your vegetables as well.

MUSTARD, YELLOW
3 teaspoons

Calories	11
Protein	0.7 gm
Carbohydrate	1.0 gm
Fat	0.7 gm
Cholesterol	0 mg
Dietary Fiber	0.4 gm

 MUSTARD GREENS

Mustard greens are the leafy part of the plant that produces mustard seeds. As members of the crucifer family of vegetables, mustard greens contain the cancer-fighting indoles.

Mustard Greens' Healing Properties

Mustard greens are superlative sources of niacin. They also contain vitamin C, beta-carotene, magnesium, iron, and calcium.

Just ½ cup of chopped, raw mustard greens contains over 250 percent of the RDA for niacin, a B-vitamin which lowers the total cholesterol, while raising the good cholesterol in many cases. So powerful are niacin's cholesterol-lowering properties that an article in the *Journal of the American Medical Association* recommended the vitamin as the "first drug to be used" in cases where simply changing the diet does not bring down the bad cholesterol.

Both beta-carotene and vitamin C in mustard greens assist niacin in preventing heart disease by controlling the oxidation reactions that can convert LDL cholesterol into its more dangerous form, making it even more likely than usual to deposit cholesterol on the artery walls. Beta-carotene and C also strengthen the immune system, and protect the body from the aging and cancer-causing effects of oxidation.

Including the Food in Your Diet

This little-noticed member of the crucifer family should be a regular addition to the diet, chopped up and added to salads. You can also sauté mustard greens in a small amount of oil, butter, or margarine.

MUSTARD GREENS
½ cup chopped, raw

Calories	7
Protein	0.8 gm
Carbohydrate	1.4 gm
Fat	0.1 gm
Cholesterol	0 mg
Dietary Fiber	0.2 gm

	Amount	RDA
Niacin	52.5 mg	263%
Vitamin C	19.6	33%
Vitamin A	148 RE	15%
Calcium	29 mg	2%
Magnesium	9 mg	2%

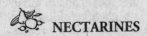 NECTARINES

A cousin to the peach, nectarines may have been named after *nektar,* the heavenly fluid that the gods of ancient Greece drank atop Mount Olympus.

The Nectarine's Healing Properties

Nectarines contain good amounts of beta-carotene and vitamin C, plus fiber, niacin, potassium, and other nutrients such as flavonoids. The beta-carotene and vitamin C in nectarines energize the immune system and help to ward off cancer. The flavonoids, pigments which give the fruit their orange color, enhance the body's ability to respond to viruses, carcinogens, and allergens. Flavonoids also strengthen collagen, the protein that holds body tissues together, and help to control damaging free radicals. The fiber in nectarines helps to prevent several types of cancer, as well as constipation.

Including the Food in Your Diet

When they are in season, eat a couple of nectarines a week. They're delicious all by themselves, in fruit salads, or even finely chopped and added to green salads.

NECTARINE
1 raw (approx. 4.8 oz)

Calories	67	
Protein	1.3 gm	
Carbohydrate	16.1 gm	
Fat	0.7 gm	
Cholesterol	0 mg	
Dietary Fiber	2.4 gm	

	Amount	RDA
Vitamin C	7.3 mg	12%
Vitamin A	100 RE	10%
Niacin	1.4 mg	7%
Potassium	288 mg	NA

 NUTS

Walnuts, hazelnuts, and chestnuts are apparently native to both the Old World and the New, suggesting that nut-bearing trees may have been growing before the continents split apart tens of millions of years ago. We do know that nuts have been cultivated for some 12,000 years.

Acorns have been eaten by many cultures the world over, and both acorns and chestnuts have been used like grains to make cereals and "mushes." The ancient Greeks must have adored acorns: their legends state that during the "Golden Age" of man, people lived primarily on this kind of nut.

There's a bit of confusion surrounding nuts, not all of which deserve the title. Technically speaking, nuts are single-seeded fruits with dry, tough fruit layers (rather than succulent ones). This means that only acorns, hazelnuts, and beechnuts are, properly speaking, nuts. The cashew is a close cousin of poison ivy, and oil from the cashew shell has been used to lubricate rocket ships. And the popular peanut is really a seed from a bush, not a nut at all.

The Nut's Healing Properties

Nuts as we know them are good sources of fiber, B-vitamins, and magnesium. The B-vitamins in nuts help to keep the brain and nervous system healthy, while the magnesium protects the heart and prevents cancer. Although nuts are generally high in fat, the fat tends to be mono or polyunsaturated fat that can help to keep cholesterol levels down. Nuts contain nutrients and phytochemicals which may help to:

• Ward off cancer
• Reduce the risk of heart disease
• Strengthen the bones
• Sharpen the mind

Nuts help to keep blood sugar under control. They also have estrogen-like properties which may help to "soften" the symptoms of menopause. Although nuts, like seeds, tend to be high in fat, eating nuts and seeds does not necessarily make one overweight. In fact, a study of over 26,000 people found that those who ate the most nuts were actually less likely to be obese, possibly because nuts are filling.

What Scientists Have Learned About Nuts

Nuts and Cancer: Nuts contain protease inhibitors which interfere with enzymes that encourage the growth of cancer. The protease inhibitors also have antioxidant properties, helping to stem the potentially cancer-causing effects of oxidation. Walnuts contain oleic acid and ellagic acid, two antioxidants that may help to protect the body against cancer. Brazil nuts have generous amounts of the mineral selenium, an antioxidant associated with lower risks of cancer.

Nuts and the Heart: Almonds and walnuts are high in monounsaturated fatty acids, the type of fat that can actually help to reduce blood cholesterol. In fact, in two different studies, supplementing the diet with almonds or walnuts drove total cholesterol levels down by 15 percent or more.

Nuts, Bones, and the Brain: Almonds, peanuts, and hazelnuts contain the mineral boron. Boron plays a vital role in keeping the bones healthy and the joints free of arthritis, for boron helps to keep calcium inside the body. Boron also plays an important role in mental alertness. People eating boron-deficient diets tend to perform poorly on simple tasks such as handling a computer joystick or picking out specific letters of the alphabet. These problems clear up when the subjects are given boron supplements.

A Brief Look at the Many Nuts

Almonds, which are related to peaches, are good sources of fiber, as well as magnesium, riboflavin, and iron.

Brazil nuts are sources of fiber, thiamin, magnesium, iron, and ellagic acid.

Cashews, which are related to poison ivy, contain magnesium, iron, zinc, and folic acid.

Chestnuts are extremely low in fat, and are good sources of fiber, vitamin C, and folic acid.

Filberts contain fiber, magnesium, and folic acid.

Hickory nuts, when dried, are good sources of fiber, thiamin, and magnesium.

Macadamia nuts, named for John Macadam of Australia, are high in fat and calories, but contain iron, magnesium, and thiamin.

Peanuts, which are actually legumes, not nuts, contain fiber, folic acid, niacin, and magnesium.

Dried pine nuts, or pignolis, are good sources of fiber, iron, magnesium, and thiamin.

Pistachio nuts are high in fiber, and contain lesser amounts of iron, thiamin, and magnesium.

Walnuts are good sources of fiber, magnesium, and folic acid.

Including the Food in Your Diet

Think of nuts as a delicious substitute for small amounts of meat, cheese, or other fatty foods. Rather than eating handfuls of nuts by themselves, add small amounts of nuts to green salads, fruit salads, vegetable and pasta dishes. Chopped nuts are also tasty additions to rice and rice dishes.

> *Caution: There is some evidence that nuts, which are relatively high in the amino acid arginine, may cause flareups of herpes. Just to be sure, some doctors advise their herpes patients to avoid nuts.*

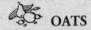 **OATS**

Oats have often been used as a laxative, an antidepressant, and a general tonic. But although oats have long been a dietary staple in many countries, it was not until the late 1970s that they began to acquire an almost mystical reputation for their seemingly phenomenal ability to lower cholesterol.

Oats' and Oat Bran's Healing Properties

Studies conducted at research centers around the world have shown that oats and oat bran may help to:

- Lower cholesterol
- Reduce the risk of certain cancers
- Relieve constipation
- Regulate blood sugar
- Possibly reduce the urge for nicotine

What Scientists Have Learned About Oats and Oat Bran

Oats and Cholesterol: Oat bran is rich in soluble fiber (which helps to drive down cholesterol levels), as well as the cholesterol-fighting substance called tocotrienol.

In a 1988 study, cholesterol levels fell in two groups of people who were following the American Heart Association's dietary guidelines. However, those who had added 2 ounces of oatmeal per day to their diets enjoyed a greater drop. The researchers found that the greatest results occurred in those who had the highest cholesterols to begin with.

How much can oat bran lower cholesterol? A study conducted at the University of Kentucky College of Medicine found that adding relatively large amounts of oat bran to the diet knocked the total cholesterol down by 12 percent or more. In other studies, cholesterol only fell by 5 or 6 percent. A 12 percent reduction in cholesterol is certainly better than a 5 percent drop, but remember that for every 1 point drop in cholesterol, the risk of heart disease falls by 2 percent. Thus, even a 5 percent reduction of cholesterol will lower the risk of heart disease by 10 percent. In some studies, heart patients were able to decrease the amounts of medicine they needed, or eliminate the drugs altogether, when they adopted a diet high in oats.

Oatmeal and oat bran both lower total cholesterol, but oat bran is perhaps twice as effective as the whole oats. Oat bran also lowers bad cholesterol while raising good. Although a 1990 study in the *Journal of the American Medical Association* reported that oat bran was no more effective at lowering cholesterol than white bread, later studies confirmed oat bran's effectiveness at lowering cholesterol. Although oat bran is not the panacea it was once thought to be, it has an important role to play in keeping cholesterol under control.

Oats and Cancer: Unlike whole wheat and wheat bran, oats and oat bran do not lower the risk of cancer by increasing the bulk of the stool and speeding it through the digestive tract. However, whole oats and oat bran contain phytates, substances which may help to control cancer by deactivating tumor-encouraging hormones.

Including the Food in Your Diet

One large bowl of oatmeal per day (or medium-sized bowl of oat bran) is enough to reduce cholesterol in most people. If you're interested in lowering your cholesterol, remember that oatmeal is only 60 to 70 percent as effective as oat bran, which is a more concentrated cholesterol-fighter.

Begin adding oat bran to your diet slowly, for it may cause gas or indigestion in some sensitive people.

OATMEAL
¾ cup, cooked

Calories	109	
Protein	4.6 gm	
Carbohydrate	19 gm	
Fat	1.8 gm	
Cholesterol	0 mg	
Dietary Fiber	3.9 gm	

	Amount	RDA
Thiamin	0.2 mg	13%
Magnesium	42 mg	11%
Iron	1.2 mg	8%

```
                    OAT BRAN
                2 tablespoons, raw

   Calories          29
   Protein           2.0 gm
   Carbohydrate      7.7 gm
   Fat               0.8 gm
   Cholesterol       0   mg
   Dietary Fiber     1.8 gm

                      Amount           RDA
   Thiamin           0.1 mg           67%
   Magnesium         27.2 mg           7%
```

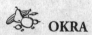 OKRA

This undervalued vegetable, which is related to the cotton plant, was grown by the Egyptians as early as A.D. 1100, and was planted in the gardens of the palace at Versailles by the French King Louis XIV. It was brought to the United States by slave traders in the 1700s, and has since been popular in the southern states. It is also enjoyed in South America, Africa, the Middle East, India, and the Caribbean.

Okra's Healing Properties

Just a ½ cup serving of sliced okra provides over 20 percent of the RDA for C, and 18 percent of the RDA for folic acid.

The same ½ cup of okra contains 2.6 grams of dietary fiber, which helps to keep blood sugar under control, reduces the risk of constipation, and offers protection against cancers of the colon, rectum, pancreas, prostate, and breast.

Including the Food in Your Diet

Surprisingly nutritious for such an overlooked vegetable, okra is delicious eaten raw. It can be chopped and added to vegetables, steamed and eaten alone, or added to many recipes. Several servings of okra per week will strengthen your immune system and improve your overall health.

OKRA
½ **cup sliced, cooked**

Calories	25	
Protein	1.5 gm	
Carbohydrate	5.8 gm	
Fat	0.1 gm	
Cholesterol	0 mg	
Dietary Fiber	2.6 gm	
	Amount	RDA
Vitamin C	13.1 mg	22%
Folacin	36.5 mcg	18%
Magnesium	46 mg	12%
Calcium	50 mg	4%
Iron	0.4 mg	2%
Potassium	257 mg	NA

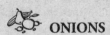 ONIONS

Onions are said to have risen from Satan's footprints as he fled the Garden of Eden, but written records regarding onions only date back to about 2400 B.C. Lower-class citizens in the Greek and Roman empires ate onions, as did Olympic athletes in training. Roman gladiators kept their muscles taut by massaging them with onion oil. During the Middle Ages, onions were used to treat bites, stings, and skin problems.

The Onion's Healing Properties

There are hundreds of members of the onion family, including red onions, white onions, scallions, leeks, shallots, and garlic. The onion has been carefully studied and a great deal of research suggests that it may:

- Thin the blood
- Lower total cholesterol
- Raise the HDL
- Reduce the risk of heart disease
- Fight cancer
- Ease breathing difficulties

Onions may help the body resist infections and lower the blood sugar. The quercetin in onions may serve as a mild sedative (in addition to being a cancer-fighting antioxidant).

What Scientists Have Learned About the Onion

Onion and Heart Disease: Eating about ½ raw onion per day can push the good cholesterol (HDL) up by as much as 25 to 30 percent in many people. HDL acts like a garbage truck, carrying bad cholesterol away from the artery walls and to the liver for disposal.

Onions contain adenosine, so they also help to keep the heart healthy by thinning the blood. Many heart attacks are triggered when a blood clot lodges in an already narrowed coronary artery, stopping the flow of blood through these vital pathways which feed the heart muscle.

Onion and Cancer: Onions contain quercetin, an antioxidant flavonoid that can disarm many potential cancer-causing agents.

Evidence of the onion's anticancer prowess was bolstered in 1994, when Japanese researchers found four anthocyanins in the red onion. Like quercetin, anthocyanins are powerful antioxidants that help the body fight off cancer. Onions contain other compounds, some based on sulfur, that slow the formation of cancer cells in the laboratory. A National Cancer Institute study has found that eating three ounces of scallions, other onions, or garlic a day can lower the risk of stomach cancer by 40 percent.

Onions and Asthma: Onions contain diphenylthiosulfinate and other substances that help to reduce the bronchial inflammation that can make breathing difficult. Other factors in onions act as antihistamines. Histamines, which are formed during allergic and inflammatory reactions, cause the smooth muscles surrounding the breathing tubes to constrict. The muscles "squeeze down" on the breathing tubes, making breathing more difficult. Onions and other foods with antihistamine properties help to relax these muscles and improve the flow of air.

Including the Food in Your Diet

Half an onion a day is enough to lower the risk of heart disease and cancer. Onions are easy to chop and add to salads, stir-fries, and many recipes. Since recipes are often designed for the faint of palate, try adding more onions than are called for.

ONION		
1 medium, raw		
Calories	38	
Protein	1.5 gm	
Carbohydrate	8.7 gm	
Fat	0.1 gm	
Cholesterol	0 mg	
Dietary Fiber	0.6 gm	
	Amount	RDA
Vitamin C	10 mg	18%

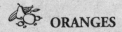

ORANGES

Oranges are believed to be natives of Southeast Asia, and were brought to the New World by Columbus. The third most popular fruit in the United States, oranges are celebrated for their vitamin C. Actually, several other foods contain more vitamin C, but because of its popularity the orange is the single most important source of the vitamin in the American diet.

The Orange's Healing Properties

Oranges are superb sources of vitamin C. They also contain lesser amounts of folic acid, thiamin, niacin, calcium, potassium, and magnesium. Oranges may:

- Reduce the risk of certain cancers
- Lower cholesterol
- Have antiviral properties
- Energize tired sperm

In addition, the flavonoids in oranges increase the body's resistance to viruses, carcinogens, and allergens, while strengthening the collagen protein which holds together body tissue.

What Scientists Have Learned About the Orange

Oranges and Cancer: A typical orange contains close to 70 mg of vitamin C, enough to imbue it with powerful anticancer properties. Various studies have shown that people who eat the most oranges tend to suffer from less cancer than those eating the fewest oranges.

But something else besides the vitamin C in the orange fights cancer. Studies have shown that while 1000 mg of supplemental vitamin C guard against cancer, three fluid ounces of orange juice a day is even more effective—but the juice contains less than 40 mg of C. Other factors in orange juice were better shields against cancer than 1000 mg of C alone. These extra cancer-fighting substances in oranges include beta-carotene, flavonoids, terpenes, carotenoids, and the antioxidant glutathione. Orange juice was put to the cancer test when laboratory animals were exposed to a known carcinogen and given the equivalent of a gallon of orange juice a day. The test animals developed 40 percent fewer signs of cancer than expected if they had not been given the orange juice.

Oranges and Cholesterol: Pectin, a soluble fiber found in the orange's membranes and skin, helps to lower cholesterol. Various studies with pectin have found that this fiber can lower total cholesterol, while raising HDL ("good") cholesterol.

Oranges and Sperm: The sperm of a young man tends to be healthier, more active, and less likely to clump together than the sperm of an older man. Animal studies suggest that vitamin C helps to keep sperm "young," active, and effective.

A researcher at the University of Texas Medical Branch in Galveston, Texas, gave daily doses of 100 mg vitamin C to men who were having difficulty getting their wives pregnant. When given C, their sperm counts jumped up, and the individual sperm were healthier and more active. Within two months, all of the men who were receiving vitamin C impregnated their wives. (Men in the control group, who were not getting the vitamin C, did not enjoy such success.) Later studies found that doses as low as 200 mg of C a day, the amount one could get from eating four oranges, could restore sperm's health and activity.

Including the Food in Your Diet

An orange a day may be as effective at keeping the doctor away as a daily apple. The amount of vitamin C in a single orange was more than enough to hold cancer at bay—and that's not even taking into account the orange's other cancer-fighting phytochemicals.

ORANGE
1 raw (approx. 4.6 oz)

Calories	62	
Protein	1.3 gm	
Carbohydrate	15.4 gm	
Fat	0.2 gm	
Cholesterol	0 mg	
Dietary Fiber	3.0 gm	
	Amount	RDA
Vitamin C	69.7 mg	116%
Folacin	39.7 mcg	20%
Thiamin	0.2 mg	13%
Calcium	52 mg	4%
Potassium	237 mg	NA

 OYSTERS

Not too many years ago, if you listened in as older men spoke in hushed voices, you might hear them talking about oysters. "Eastern oysters," one would say to the others. "The Eastern oysters will do it." They were referring to the oyster's reputed ability to aid men who were having sexual difficulties, especially oysters from the Atlantic Ocean. But what they were discussing was nothing new, for the oyster's reputation as an aphrodisiac and an aid to impotent men is ancient.

The Oyster's Healing Properties

Oysters contain enormous amounts of zinc, as well as iron and vitamins A, C, and B_{12}. Oysters may help to:

- Aid men's sexuality and potency
- Protect against overgrowth of the prostate
- Strengthen the immune system

- Prevent memory degeneration
- Reduce the risk of heart disease and stroke

The zinc in oysters may also help to prevent vision loss with aging, because it protects a part of the retina called the macula. Oysters also contain copper, which may act as a natural pain-killer.

What Scientists Have Learned About Oysters

Oysters, Sex, and Reproduction: Male potency and sperm formation depend upon adequate amounts of zinc in the body. If you put men on a zinc-deficient diet, their sperm counts will fall slightly.

If low zinc causes low sperm counts, will zinc supplements make infertile men fertile again? Fourteen infertile men in India, ranging in age from 24 to 45, were given zinc supplements. Four months later, their sperm counts were significantly higher, and individual sperm moved about with increased energy. Best of all, two of the men's wives were already pregnant. Three ounces of oysters contain a whopping 456 percent of the RDA for zinc (68 mg), more than enough to interest men in the little sea creature's potency-potentiating properties.

Oysters and the Prostate: Zinc is also essential for a healthy prostate, that little gland that plays such a major role in male sexual performance. The prostate gland, which sits right below a man's bladder and is wrapped around the urethra, has a greater concentration of zinc than any other organ in the body.

Many men begin to suffer from BPH (benign prostatic hypertrophy) in their fifties or sixties. With BPH the prostate grows, often clamping down on the urethra. Since urine in the bladder has to pass through the urethra in order to exit the body, problems can occur when the prostate squeezes on this vital tube. BPH can cause straining to urinate, dribbling, urgency, and having to get up to urinate many times during the night.

Fortunately, BPH symptoms can sometimes be reduced by giving men zinc supplements. In one study discussed at the 1974 meeting of the American Medical Association in Chicago, 19 patients who had been given zinc enjoyed a reduction in their BPH symptoms. X-rays and other studies also showed that the prostates of 14 of those men had shrunk.

Oysters and the Immune System: Zinc plays a major role in keeping the immune system strong. A lack of zinc can cause the thymus gland (the "school" for immune-system cells) to shrink. When the thymus gland shrivels, there are fewer T-cells available to fight off "germs" inside the body. T-cell levels normally fall with age. But when Italian researchers gave 15 mg of zinc to elderly subjects, their T-cell levels jumped up to match the levels found in young people. (The B-cells that play a vital role in our body's ability to "remember" and fight off diseases also need zinc.)

Zinc helps the body resist disease in another way, by slowing the growth of certain bacteria which cause disease. It may also help to control the bacteria which cause tooth decay, and lessen the symptoms of a cold. In a 1987 study, 57 volunteers were given zinc supplements and exposed to a cold virus. Compared to a control group that received a placebo, the zinc group had significantly fewer cold symptoms. In the same study, 69 people were actually injected with a cold virus. Those who then developed a cold were given either zinc or a placebo. Again, the zinc group suffered much less than did the placebo group.

Oysters and Memory: Healthy people who are deliberately given a zinc-deficient diet will begin to develop trouble with their short-term memories, and will have difficulty performing various mental tasks. Although it does not appear that taking large amounts of zinc will make one "super-smart," it is clear that getting at least the minimal amounts spelled out in the RDAs will help to keep the brain sharp. A single ounce of raw oysters supplies much more than the RDA for zinc, so oysters are a good "brain food."

Oysters, the Heart, and Strokes: Oysters contain the omega-3 fatty acids which protect the heart by lowering LDL cholesterol and raising HDL cholesterol. The omega-3s also help to thin the blood and prevent unnecessary blood clots, which can cause heart attacks and strokes.

Including the Food in Your Diet

Occasionally enjoying cooked oysters will provide you with a great deal of zinc, as well as iron and other nutrients. Make sure that you eat cooked, not raw oysters. Each oyster filters up to 25 gallons of water a day through its body. If the oyster is from polluted waters (and so many waters are polluted these days) there is an excellent chance that the oyster contains harmful bacteria or other organisms.

OYSTERS
3 oz, baked or broiled

Calories	133	
Protein	8.9 gm	
Carbohydrate	9.8 gm	
Fat	6.2 gm	
Cholesterol	45.9 mg	
Dietary Fiber	0.1 gm	
	Amount	RDA
Zinc	68.4 mg	456%
Iron	5.4 mg	36%
Vitamin A	136.7 RE	14%
Niacin	2.6 mg	13%
Calcium	99.9 mg	8%

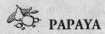 **PAPAYA**

The exact origin of the tropical papaya is not known, although it is probably native to the Americas. Most markets in the United States sell the familiar Solo papaya, although the longer Mexican varieties can be found in ethnic grocery stores. Papaya has been used to treat diarrhea, allergies, hay fever, indigestion, and other ailments.

The Papaya's Healing Properties

Papaya is a superlative source of vitamin C, with an average papaya providing over 300 percent of the RDA for this vitamin. Good amounts of C help to keep oxidation damage under control, ward off cancer and heart disease, and strengthen the immune system. Papaya also contains excellent amounts of beta-carotene. Like vitamin C, beta-carotene acts as an anti-oxidant to protect the heart and hold cancer at bay. Beta-carotene also plays an important role in growth, sleep, vision, skin health, and the health of the immune system.

Papaya contains an enzyme called papain, which helps the body to digest proteins. Papaya fruit and papaya juice are traditional remedies for indigestion. More recently, "papaya pills" have been used for the same purpose.

Including the Food in Your Diet

With three times the RDA for vitamin C, and more than half the allowance of beta-carotene, a single papaya is quite a health booster. Enjoy one several times a week when it is in season, alone, in a fruit salad, or as a side dish. It's delicious with a little bit of lime juice sprinkled on top.

PAPAYA
1 raw (approx. 11 oz)

Calories	120	
Protein	2.0 gm	
Carbohydrate	30.0 gm	
Fat	0.5 gm	
Cholesterol	0 mg	
Dietary Fiber	2.9 gm	

	Amount		RDA
Vitamin C	190	mg	317%
Vitamin A	615	RE	62%
Calcium	75	mg	6%
Potassium	790	mg	NA

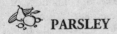 **PARSLEY**

Parsley is the Rodney Dangerfield of foods. This herb receives little respect, despite the fact that it is surprisingly nutritious! Ounce for ounce, it has more beta-carotene than broccoli or spinach, more vitamin C than carrots, spinach, or sweet potatoes, and good amounts of potassium and calcium.

Parsley's Healing Properties

The little sprig of parsley shoved to the side of most dinner plates has powerful medicinal properties. It contains several anticancer ingredients, including vitamin C, beta-carotene, chlorophyll, flavonoids, polyacetylenes, coumarins, and monoterpenes.

Vitamin C, beta-carotene, monoterpenes, and some of the flavonoids are antioxidants that help to control the damage caused by oxidation. Oxidation damage can lead to cancer of the lung and other cancers. The polyacetylenes in parsley work to reduce the risk of cancer by inhibiting the production of prostaglandins, substances which, under certain circumstances, might encourage the growth of cancer.

Parsley is a particularly rich source of chlorophyll, a plant pigment that has been called "nature's natural cleanser" for its prowess in reducing body, urinary, and fecal odor, as well as its ability to fight off cancer and the cancer-causing effects of oxidation.

Including the Food in Your Diet

Low in calories but high in vitamin C and folacin, parsley should be a regular addition to the dinner plate. But don't toss the parsley sprig aside—eat it. Not only does it taste good, it's an effective breath freshener.

PARSLEY
½ cup chopped, raw

Calories	10	
Protein	0.7 gm	
Carbohydrate	2.1 gm	
Fat	0.1 gm	
Cholesterol	0 mg	
Dietary Fiber	——	

	Amount	RDA
Vitamin C	27 mg	45%
Folacin	55 mcg	28%
Vitamin A	156 RE	16%
Iron	1.9 mg	13%

 PARSNIPS

Cousin to the carrot, this Eurasian native was eaten by the Ancient Greeks and Romans. The modern variety of the parsnip was developed during Medieval times. The vegetable was a mainstay of the Colonial American and European diets until replaced by potatoes a few hundred years ago.

The Parsnip's Healing Properties

Although it looks like a light-brown version of the carrot, and is related to the carrot, parsnips do not have beta-carotene. Parsnips contain very good amounts of vitamin C and folic acid, plus vitamin E, complex carbohydrates, and fiber.

Including the Food in Your Diet

Eat as many as you like, adding them to stews, casseroles, and other dishes. At least one or two servings a week will help to maintain good health.

> ### PARSNIPS
> #### ½ cup slices, cooked
>
> | | | |
> |---|---|---|
> | Calories | 63 | |
> | Protein | 1.0 gm | |
> | Carbohydrate | 15.2 gm | |
> | Fat | 0.2 gm | |
> | Cholesterol | 0 mg | |
> | Dietary Fiber | 2.1 gm | |
>
> | | Amount | RDA |
> |---|---|---|
> | Folacin | 45.4 mcg | 23% |
> | Vitamin C | 10.1 mg | 17% |
> | Magnesium | 23 mg | 6% |
> | Potassium | 287 mg | NA |

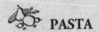 PASTA

Although legend tells us that Marco Polo was introduced to noodles during his travels to China and brought them back to Italy in 1295, inhabitants of the Italian peninsula were making pasta as early as 400 B.C.

There are many types of pasta, which means "paste" in Italian. The best for your health, of course, is pasta made from whole-wheat flour.

Pasta's Healing Properties

Thanks to its large concentration of complex carbohydrates, plus its thiamin and fiber, fresh pasta may:

- Act as a stress-reducer and sleep aid
- Reduce the risk of heart disease
- Fight cancer

What Scientists Have Learned About Pasta

Pasta, Sleep, and Depression: Scientific evidence suggests that the amino acid tryptophan helps people to sleep and relieves some forms of depression. But first, the tryptophan must reach the brain.

Many foods contain tryptophan, but this amino acid cannot simply ''stroll'' into the brain. Instead, it must find a ''seat'' on the carriers that transport amino acids. But trytophan must compete for ''seats'' with five other amino acids. Since it does not compete very well, it is difficult for large amounts of tryptophan to reach the brain.

Carbohydrate-rich meals increase the production of insulin which, in turn, effectively reduces the levels of the other five amino acids in the blood. This makes it easier for tryptophan to find a ''seat'' and be transported into the brain. (High-protein meals have the opposite effect.) Once inside the brain, tryptophan can be converted into a neurotransmitter called serotonin, which aids in sleep, elevates the mood, and regulates appetite. Thus pasta, like a glass of milk, may be a good night-time food to help one to sleep.

Pasta, Heart Disease, and Cancer: The complex carbohydrates and fiber in pasta help to reduce the risk of heart disease by lowering both the total cholesterol and the LDL (''bad'') cholesterol. Every little bit helps with heart disease: a 1-point drop in total cholesterol lowers the risk of heart disease by 2 percent. Pasta's fiber also guards against cancers of the colon and rectum. Keep in mind that whole-wheat pasta has more than double the fiber of regular pasta.

Including the Food in Your Diet

Several helpings of pasta per week will help to protect your heart and promote good general health. If you eat it with tomato sauce, you'll also be getting lots of the powerful antioxidant called lycopene.

```
                         PASTA
                 1 cup spaghetti, cooked

   Calories              197
   Protein               6.7 gm
   Carbohydrate          39.7 gm
   Fat                   .9 gm
   Cholesterol           0   mg
   Dietary Fiber         3.1 gm

                         Amount            RDA
   Thiamin               0.2 mg            13%
   Iron                  1.7 mg            11%
   Niacin                1.5 mg             8%
```

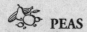 **PEAS**

> *Eat peas with the king and cherries with*
> *the beggar.* —ENGLISH PROVERB

No one knows exactly where the pea originated, although the oldest known pea, dating back to 9700 B.C., was found in Southeast Asia. Pea soup was sold in the streets of ancient Rome, and peas became a fad at the court of France's King Louis XIV: both his wife and his mistress loved eating peas. English men and women of the Middle Ages and later times called peas "pease," and their children recited the rhyme "Pease porridge hot, pease porridge cold . . ." A monk named Gregor Mendel put the pea in the scientific literature when he used it to perform his groundbreaking experiments in genetics.

The Pea's Healing Properties

Peas, which are low in fat, contain vitamins B$_6$ and C, niacin, thiamin, folic acid, iron, and magnesium. Just ½ cup of cooked peas contains 25 percent of the RDA for niacin, a B-family vitamin which helps to combat arthritis, asthma, and cancer, while controlling cholesterol. The same amount of peas also provides 3 grams of dietary fiber, plus the antioxidant, cancer-fighting flavonoids.

Including the Food in Your Diet

Although there is no ''RDA'' for legumes such as peas, it is clear that they are low-fat bundles of nutrition that make a tasty addition to any dietary plan. They can be eaten steamed or boiled, as a side dish, or added to various dishes. They're also surprisingly tasty, although a little ''sharp'' in flavor, when sprouted. Several servings of peas a week will help to keep your heart healthy.

PEAS
½ cup, cooked

Calories	67	
Protein	4.3 gm	
Carbohydrate	12.5 gm	
Fat	0.2 gm	
Cholesterol	0 mg	
Dietary Fiber	3.0 gm	

	Amount	RDA
Folacin	50.7 mcg	25%
Vitamin C	11.4 mg	19%
Magnesium	31 mg	8%
Potassium	217 mg	NA

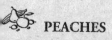

PEACHES

Although the peach is not native to the United States, it was so widely planted across the eastern seaboard by early settlers that many Colonial botanists thought that the fruit was indigenous.

The third most popular of all fruits grown in the United States, the peach comes in many varieties, including the "Elegant Lady," "Red Top," "Flavor Crest," and "Rio Oso Gem." Most of the peaches purchased fresh in markets are soft, juicy freestone peaches, with pits that detach easily from the flesh. Canned peaches tend to be "clingstone," meaning that the flesh and pit are harder to separate.

The Peach's Healing Properties

The sweet-tasting, low-calorie peach is high in beta-carotene, vitamin C, boron and fiber. It's also low in fat and sodium, and has no cholesterol. One raw peach contains 47 percent of the RDA for beta-carotene. Beta-carotene is a powerful antioxidant which strengthens the immune system, enhances the body's ability to fight infection, and protects the eyes against oxidative damage which can dim or destroy vision. The boron in peaches helps to keep the bones strong and the memory sharp. Peaches also have mild laxative properties, as do other fruits, due to the fiber content.

Including the Food in Your Diet

The Food & Nutrition Board recommends five or more servings of fruits and vegetables a day. Eating a peach a day, when they are in season, is a tasty way to work toward this goal.

Fresh peaches contain the highest amounts of nutrients and fiber. If you eat canned peaches, choose peaches canned in their own juice, not swimming in sugary syrup.

PEACH
1 raw (approx. 4 oz)

Calories	37
Protein	0.7 gm
Carbohydrate	9.7 gm
Fat	0.1 gm
Cholesterol	0 mg
Dietary Fiber	0.6 gm

	Amount	RDA
Vitamin A	465 IU	47%
Vitamin C	5.7 mg	10%

 PEARS

No pear falls into a shut mouth.
—ITALIAN PROVERB

First cultivated as early as 2000 B.C., the pear remains a popular fruit today. Although several thousand varieties of pear have been developed, commercial growers produce just over one hundred varieties.

The Pear's Healing Properties

Low in calories and fat, pears are good sources of fiber. They also contain vitamin C, folic acid, potassium, and boron.

In addition, pears contain pectin, a soluble fiber which helps to lower cholesterol. In a study of 27 patients, taking pectin for eight weeks drove cholesterol down by over more than 7 percent, which reduces the risk of heart disease by 14 percent. (Remember, every 1 point drop in total cholesterol reduces the risk of coronary heart disease by 2 percent.) The pectin also cut the harmful LDL cholesterol by 10 percent.

The boron in pears is perhaps as important as calcium for

keeping bones strong. Calcium is needed to build bones, but boron acts as a policeman to keep calcium from "escaping" the body and weakening the bones. Even if a diet is high in calcium, there must also be good supplies of boron to make sure that the calcium behaves itself and stays where it belongs. Boron also helps to keep the brain sharp. When volunteers were deliberately placed on a boron-deficient diet, their mental acuity diminished measurably. Replacing the boron solved the problem.

Including the Food in Your Diet

With its carbohydrates, pectin, vitamin C, boron, and other nutrients, the pear should be eaten often when in season. A fresh pear a day, or pear slices in yogurt, are a medicinal addition to the diet. Be sure to eat the pear skin; that's where most of the vitamin C is located.

PEAR
1 raw (approx. 6.0 oz)

Calories	98	
Protein	0.7 gm	
Carbohydrate	25.1 gm	
Fat	0.7 gm	
Cholesterol	0 mg	
Dietary Fiber	4.2 gm	
	Amount	RDA
Vitamin C	6.6 mg	11%
Folacin	12.1 mcg	6%
Potassium	208 mg	NA

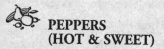

PEPPERS
(HOT & SWEET)

Peppers have long been regarded as a medicine. The ancient Mayans used peppers for pain, coughs, sore throats, asthma, and other respiratory ailments. Europeans of the 1600s felt that peppers cured digestive problems and ulcers—and modern evidence backs them up. In more recent times, peppers have been put into heating liniments to soothe sore muscles, used as a cure for toothaches, and made into an anti-inflammatory preparation for the eye. They have also been used as aphrodisiacs: As early as the sixteenth century, priests were warned that peppers made one overly lustful.

Peppers have also been good for the health of at least one entire city. Jesse James is said to have refrained from robbing the bank in McKinney, Texas, because he liked the chili served at the McKinney saloon. (Their chili was full of peppers.)

The vegetable we call a pepper is not the same as the black pepper that we sprinkle on our food. Green peppers, red peppers, chili peppers, and the like, which are native to the New World, are not related to peppercorn, an Asian native which is ground up to make black pepper, a condiment.

The Pepper's Healing Properties

Bell, banana, cubanelle, and pimiento peppers are sweet peppers. Anaheim, ancho, cascabel, cayenne, cherry, habañero, Hungarian wax, jalapeño, poblano, and serrano peppers are hot peppers. Studies show that peppers may help to:

• Relieve pain
• Reduce symptoms of the cold and other respiratory ailments
• Lower the risk of heart attack and stroke
• Fight cancer

Like garlic and ginger, chili peppers are clot busters that help to prevent heart attacks, strokes, and retinal degeneration due to blood clots by keeping the blood thin. Chili peppers may also help to keep the waistline trim by speeding up the metabolism and encouraging the body to burn calories.

What Scientists Have Learned About Peppers

Hot Chili Peppers and Pain: Capsaicin, the substance that makes chili peppers hot, is used in an ointment called Zostrix to relieve arthritis and shingles pain. The capsaicin seems to work by rapidly "burning out" certain nerve cells, rendering them incapable of passing along pain signals. Even though the painful stimulus may still be present, the pain "message" can't get through.

Eating hot peppers also stimulates the release of endorphins, the pain-blocking hormones first discovered in the 1970s. Like capsaicin, the endorphins block pain signals traveling through the nervous system, thus relieving the pain. Endorphins also "lift" the mood, giving one an overall sense of well-being.

Hot Peppers, the Nose, and the Lungs: Like garlic and other spicy foods, hot peppers can "wash out" the respiratory system, flushing away mucus clogging the bronchial tubes. Mucus, which is normally moist and soft and easily swept through the respiratory system, is troublesome if it becomes hard and sticky. The irritation caused by eating hot peppers causes the body to release fluid into the respiratory system (nasal passages, throat, and bronchial tubes). These fluids help wash away lodged mucus and make breathing easier.

In addition, the vitamin C in peppers acts as an antihistamine to ease breathing. The Second National Health & Nutrition Examination Survey found that people with higher vitamin C intakes (200 mg more per day) had only two-thirds as much bronchitis and wheezing as did those getting lesser amounts of C.

Hot Peppers, Heart Disease, and Cancer: Peppers as a group have more vitamin C than citrus fruits, which are mistakenly considered the best source of vitamin C. Ounce for ounce, hot peppers contain over three times the vitamin C of an orange. A single chili pepper has twice the RDA for vitamin C, and a full day's RDA for beta-carotene. Such generous supplies of these two antioxidant vitamins help the body resist the oxidation-conversion of LDL ("bad") cholesterol into its more dangerous form, a form which is more likely to leave artery-blocking deposits on the wall of the coronary arteries in the heart.

Beta-carotene and vitamin C also help the body fight cancer by reducing the oxidation damage to cellular DNA that can turn harmless cells into cancerous ones. In addition, the two nutrients strengthen the immune system in its fight against the cancers that do manage to arise within the body. Epidemiological studies, which look at large groups of people, their diets, and their diseases, have found that eating large amounts of vitamin C–rich foods protects against cancer of the esophagus, stomach, pancreas, cervix, rectum, breast, and lungs. Laboratory studies have shown that vitamin C can kill tumor cells directly, can increase the immune system's ability to destroy tumors, and can increase the effectiveness of other cancer therapies. In a study of cancer victims and radiation therapy, 50 previously untreated patients were given either radiation therapy, or radiation plus 5 grams (.18 oz) of C a day. One month later, the cancer had completely disappeared in 55 percent of the radiation-only group—and in 87 percent of the radiation-plus-C patients.

Sweet red and green peppers have additional cancer-fighting ingredients. Green peppers contain *p*-coumaric acid and chloregenic acid, two substances which bind up and carry out of the body the nitric oxides from our foods that might otherwise be converted into potentially cancer-causing nitrosamines. And red peppers contain the cancer-fighting lycopene, which is also found in tomatoes.

Including the Food in Your Diet

A daily drink of about fifteen drops of hot chili sauce mixed in water, or several spicy meals per week, can help to keep the respiratory system clear and the air flowing freely. Adding ½ cup of sliced red pepper to salads, casseroles, stir-fries, sandwiches, or other foods every day will provide enough to confer many of the vitamin's protective effects against cancer and heart disease. Eating chili peppers does not cause ulcers. If you have ulcers, however, you should not eat peppers or other foods which cause pain or other problems.

PEPPERS, GREEN BELL
½ cup chopped, raw

Calories	14
Protein	0.5 gm
Carbohydrate	3.2 gm
Fat	0.1 gm
Cholesterol	0 mg
Dietary Fiber	0.8 gm

	Amount	RDA
Vitamin C	45 mg	75%
Folacin	11 mcg	6%
Vitamin B$_6$	0.1 mcg	5%

PEPPERS, RED BELL
½ cup chopped, raw

Calories	14
Protein	0.5 gm
Carbohydrate	3.2 gm
Fat	0.1 gm
Cholesterol	0 mg
Dietary Fiber	0.8 gm

	Amount	RDA
Vitamin C	26.1 mg	44%
Vitamin B$_6$	0.7 mg	35%
Iron	2.8 mg	19%
Thiamin	0.2 mg	18%
Niacin	3.3 mg	17%
Magnesium	54.5 mg	14%
Folacin	22.2 mcg	11%
Potassium	844 mg	NA

PEPPERS, CHILI
1 Tablespoon, raw

Calories	4
Protein	0.2 gm
Carbohydrate	0.9 gm
Fat	trace
Cholesterol	0 mg
Dietary Fiber	0.1 gm

	Amount	RDA
Vitamin C	23 mg	38%
Vitamin A	101 RE	10%

 PINEAPPLES

Native to South America, pineapples created quite a stir when seafaring explorers brought them to Europe in the early 1500s. The fruit was so popular that designers of buildings and coats-of-arms incorporated it into their works. In the 1700s the pineapple was taken to Hawaii, where it took root.

The Pineapple's Healing Properties

Low in fat and calories, the pineapple contains a very good amount of vitamin C, plus fiber, B-vitamins, magnesium, and iron. In addition, the sweet yellow fruit contains lesser-known substances with strong medicinal properties: manganese, and the enzymes bromelain and peroxidase.

Manganese is a trace mineral found in only small quantities in the body. One cup of raw pineapple pieces contains 2.5 mg of manganese, enough to put one well within the "Estimated Safe and Adequate Daily Dietary Intake" of 2.0 to 5.0 mg per day.

Manganese strengthens the immune system by enhancing the activity of natural killer cells and macrophages (the giant "cell eaters" that literally engulf and destroy bacteria and other foreign substances in the body). Since manganese is an important co-factor in the enzyme systems that handle glucose (sugar), the body needs adequate supplies of the mineral in order to regulate blood sugar. Manganese deficiency can lead to glucose intolerance and the symptoms of diabetes, problems which are erased by giving manganese supplements.

Manganese may also be a boon for women suffering from abnormally long or heavy menstrual periods (menorrhagia). When fifteen women were deliberately placed on a diet low in manganese, the volume of their menstrual fluid increased by 50 percent, and they lost increased amounts of several important minerals during menstruation. This suggests that manganese helps to regulate fluid flow during menstruation, and that manganese-rich foods or manganese supplements may assist women with menorrhagia.

The bromelain and peroxidase found in pineapple are two of the many enzymes which make life possible by "speeding up" chemical reactions in the body. Since bromelain's medical value was first recognized in the late 1950s, over 200 reports in the scientific literature have discussed the enzyme's efficacy in treating angina (chest pain related to coronary artery disease), arthritis, bronchitis, burns, menstrual difficulties, swelling, digestive problems, pneumonia, infections, and other ailments. The other enzyme, peroxidase, has been identified as a tumor-fighter. And peroxidase's anticancer activity is enhanced by the presence of the antioxidant vitamin C in pineapple: A single cup of pineapple cubes provides 40 percent of the RDA for this immune-boosting, cancer-fighting vitamin.

Including the Food in Your Diet

Several servings per week of fresh pineapple, or pineapple canned in its own juice, strengthen the immune system and bones, while supplying the body with a variety of nutrients. Chopped pineapple tastes great added to salads and stir-fries.

PINEAPPLE
1 cup cubes

Calories	76	
Protein	0.6 gm	
Carbohydrate	19.2 gm	
Fat	0.7 gm	
Cholesterol	0 mg	
Dietary Fiber	1.9 gm	

	Amount	RDA
Vitamin C	23.9 mg	40%
Folacin	16.4 mcg	8%
Thiamin	0.1 mg	7%
Vitamin B_6	0.1 mg	5%
Magnesium	21.7 mg	5%
Iron	0.6 mg	4%

 PLUMS/PRUNES

The plum, native to the Caucasus region of Asia, is related to the almond. A prune is simply a dried plum, although only ''prune'' plums (those with yellow meat) make good prunes.

The Healing Properties of Plums and Prunes

Plums: This small, dark fruit is low in fat and calories. Two plums (4 to 5 ounces) contain only 70 to 80 calories. A single plum has slightly over 10 percent of the RDA for vitamin C, plus riboflavin, vitamin B_6, potassium, carotenes, and flavonoids. Plums have laxative, antibacterial, and antiviral properties.

Prunes: These dried plums are powerful laxatives, although no one is quite sure why they work. Eating about a dozen prunes a day is enough to increase the size of bowel movements by up to 20 percent. Some researchers have pointed to the prune's fiber and magnesium, but studies with fiber or magnesium alone don't explain the prune's laxative prowess. Another possibility is the prune's high concentration of a sugar called sorbitol, which has laxative properties.

The soluble fiber in prunes helps to lower total cholesterol, as well as the artery-harming LDL ("bad") cholesterol.

Including the Food in Your Diet

Enjoy fresh plums and prunes several times a week. If you are troubled by constipation, try eating a dozen or so prunes, or drinking ½ to 1 cup of prune juice daily. You can begin with smaller portions, adding a little more every day to find the amount of whole prunes or prune juice that works best for you.

Since prune juice is naturally sweet and high in calories, look for prune juice that has no added sugar.

PLUM
1 raw (approx. 2.3 oz)

Calories	36	
Protein	0.6 gm	
Carbohydrate	8.6 gm	
Fat	0.5 gm	
Cholesterol	0 mg	
Dietary Fiber	1 gm	
	Amount	RDA
Vitamin C	6.3 mg	11%
Thiamin	0.1 mg	7%
Riboflavin	0.1 mg	6%
Vitamin B$_6$	0.1 mg	5%
Potassium	113 mg	NA

PRUNE
5, dried, pitted (approx. 1.5 oz)

Calories	100	
Protein	1.1	gm
Carbohydrate	26.0	gm
Fat	0.25	gm
Cholesterol	0	mg
Dietary Fiber	3.0	gm

	Amount		RDA
Vitamin A	84	RE	8%
Iron	1.0	mg	7%
Magnesium	19	mg	5%
Potassium	313	mg	NA

 POMEGRANATES

Regarded in ancient folklore as a fertility symbol, the pomegranate is a tasty addition to the diet.

The Healing Properties of the Pomegranate

Low in fat and sodium, the pomegranate contains vitamin C, potassium, and other nutrients, including a large "dose" of fiber. The pomegranate's fiber speeds the transit of the stool rapidly through the bowels, helping to relieve constipation as well as the hemorrhoids and other ills that may be caused by straining. Fiber also helps to guard against colon and other cancers.

Including the Food in Your Diet

As an occasional snack, pomegranates make an excellent addition to a healthy diet. To eat, cut one in half, loosen the seeds with your finger and eat them. But watch out! The juice may squirt out of the seeds and stain your clothing.

POMEGRANATE
1 raw (approx. 5.5 oz)

Calories	104	
Protein	1.5 gm	
Carbohydrate	26.5 gm	
Fat	0.5 gm	
Cholesterol	0 mg	
Dietary Fiber	5.1 gm	

	Amount	RDA
Vitamin C	9.4 mg	16%
Potassium	399 mg	NA

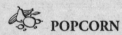 POPCORN

A native American named Quadequina introduced the early European settlers to popcorn at the first Thanksgiving feast. Popcorn quickly began a dietary staple, later evolving into a sweetened treat. A relatively plain movie and snack staple through most of the twentieth century, popcorn became a specialty and gourmet item in the 1970s, and found itself coated with or dipped in root beer, chocolate, butter rum, pineapple, and just about every other imaginable flavoring and coloring.

Popcorn's Healing Properties

Popcorn is likely the healthiest snack food around. By itself, popcorn is low in calories and fat, and has absolutely no cholesterol. Made entirely of corn, it contains folic acid, vitamin C, and fiber.

Including the Food in Your Diet

Eaten in moderation, air-popped popcorn without added butter or salt is an excellent snack and stomach-filler. Sprinkled with a little bit of garlic or onion powder, it can help to keep heart disease and cancer at bay.

```
┌─────────────────────────────────────────┐
│  ┌───────────────────────────────────┐  │
│  │            POPCORN                 │  │
│  │    1 cup unsalted, air-popped      │  │
│  │                                    │  │
│  │   Calories         23              │  │
│  │   Protein          0.8 gm          │  │
│  │   Carbohydrate     4.6 gm          │  │
│  │   Fat              0.3 gm          │  │
│  │   Cholesterol      0   mg          │  │
│  │   Dietary Fiber    0.9 gm          │  │
│  └───────────────────────────────────┘  │
└─────────────────────────────────────────┘
```

 POTATOES

The medicinal history of potatoes, which are native to Peru, is somewhat shaky. When Queen Elizabeth's cooks first prepared the exotic food for Her Majesty in the 1500s, they mistakenly threw away the odd-looking tubers (potatoes), and instead served the stems and leaves, which made the queen and her guests quite sick. (We now know that stems and leaves of potatoes contain small amounts of a poison.) In the years that followed, potatoes were blamed for causing syphilis and leprosy, as well as moral decay and laziness. The potato's fortunes rose when the French court took a fancy to the tuber in 1780.

Potatoes have a brief medicinal history. From the late 1700s to the early 1900s, they were used to treat sunburn, frostbite, black eyes, gout, rheumatism, and warts.

The Potato's Healing Properties

Potatoes as "pep" foods? Sounds strange, but potatoes are filled with vitamins and minerals that energize the mind and body. Potatoes are a good source of potassium, with a single potato providing over 800 mg of the mineral. A lack of potassium commonly leads to a generalized feeling of weakness and fatigue. In one study of senior citizens, who often have low levels of potassium, those with potassium-poor diets also had weaker-than-normal grip strengths.

A single potato also contains 14 percent of the RDA for magnesium and 11 percent of the RDA for folic acid. The mineral magnesium is essential for the synthesis of ATP (adenosinetriphosphate), a vital part of the processes which make energy available for use by the body. And a lack of energy is one of the symptoms of a folic acid deficiency. People who tire easily or who suffer from depression often see their symptoms vanish when given folic acid. Folic acid can also help to relieve "restless leg," a syndrome characterized by fatigue, itching, and twitching of the leg muscles.

Even the vitamin C in potatoes may play a role in energy and "pep." Knowing that feeling tired is one of the symptoms of a vitamin C deficiency, British researchers looked at 411 dentists and their wives. They found that the ones who got the greatest amounts of C had only half the fatigue symptoms of those who got the smallest amounts. (Incidentally, potatoes are the main source of vitamin C in the American diet. Not because they contain extraordinary amounts of the vitamin, but because so much of the vegetable is eaten: 125 pounds per person, per year.)

With all those energy-enhancing nutrients, potatoes are definitely a power food. In addition, potatoes contain protease inhibitors and polyphenols, which disarm certain cancer-causing agents and prevent the cellular mutations that can lead to cancer. The large amounts of potassium in potatoes help to keep the heartbeat regular and the blood pressure at proper levels. In fact, the level of potassium in the blood serum can be used to gauge the likelihood of suffering from irregular heartbeat (ventricular tachycardia and premature ventricular contractions) during the early stages of a heart attack. Also, higher levels of potassium in the blood suggest better odds of recovery from a heart attack.

Including the Food in Your Diet

With very good amounts of vitamins C and B_6, plus iron and potassium and other nutrients, potatoes are all-around health enhancers. Baked or mashed, they should be eaten several times a week. Enjoy potatoes plain, or with light seasoning. Drowning potatoes in heavy, fatty sauces turns a healthy, low-fat food into a danger to the heart and general health.

POTATO
1 baked, with skin and flesh
(approx. 7.1 oz)

Calories	220	
Protein	4.6 gm	
Carbohydrate	5.1 gm	
Fat	0.2 gm	
Cholesterol	0 mg	
Dietary Fiber	2.2 gm	

	Amount	RDA
Vitamin C	26.1 mg	44%
Vitamin B₆	0.7 mg	35%
Iron	2.7 mg	18%
Niacin	3.3 mg	17%
Magnesium	56 mg	14%
Thiamin	0.2 mg	13%
Folacin	22.2 mcg	11%
Potassium	844 mg	NA

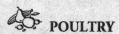 **POULTRY**

Chicken, turkey, duck, goose, partridge, pheasant, and quail are all members of the poultry family, of which chicken and turkey are the most popular. Chicken consumption got a boost in the 1940s when changes in breeding and marketing practices made the previously expensive chicken affordable to the average person. Consumption rose again in the 1970s as health-conscious people began shifting from meat to poultry. The average American now consumes about 50 pounds of chicken a year.

Although fewer turkeys are eaten, they are American natives and, if Benjamin Franklin had had his way, would have been the national bird.

Poultry's Healing Properties

Chicken: Although most cuts of chicken are relatively high in fat, they are good sources of B-vitamins, zinc, iron, magnesium, and potassium, as well as complete protein.

Chicken breast cooked without the skin is the lowest in fat, getting less than 20 percent of its calories from fat. About three ounces of chicken breast supplies close to 60 percent of the RDA for niacin, 25 percent of the vitamin B_6, as well as lesser amounts of iron, magnesium, potassium, riboflavin, vitamin B_{12}, and zinc. The B-vitamins in chicken breast enhance the body's ability to extract energy from food, are vital for the growth of new red blood cells, and are absolutely essential for a healthy nervous system.

The B-vitamins are also major supports for the immune system. Without good levels of B_6 and B_{12}, the thymus gland (where T-cells receive their disease-fighting programming) would shrink, and the number of T-cells circulating in the blood would fall.

The most nutrient-packed cut of chicken is the chicken liver. Three ounces of chicken liver contains over 800 percent of the RDA for B_{12}, 400 percent of the vitamin A, almost 90 percent of the folic acid, 70 percent of the riboflavin (B_2), and 20 to 25 percent of the B_6, C, zinc and niacin. The large amounts of folic acid may be helpful to women taking birth control pills (who often lack good amounts of this nutrient). Unfortunately, chicken liver has a few drawbacks: It gets more than 30 percent of its calories from fat, and contains over 500 mg of cholesterol per 3-ounce serving.

Turkey: As with chicken, the white meat is less fatty. Three ounces of white meat turkey (without the skin) gets only 18 percent of its calories from fat. (Dark meat turkey, by comparison, gets some 35 percent of its calories from fat.) The white meat of the turkey also supplies good amounts of zinc, niacin, and vitamin B_6, as well as lesser amounts of B_{12}, iron, magnesium, potassium, and zinc. Turkey also contains tryptophan, an amino acid which helps to induce sleep. And, of course, turkey is an excellent source of protein.

Turkey liver is the most nutrient-dense part of the turkey, supplying superlative amounts of vitamin A and B_{12}, plus folic acid. Unfortunately, turkey liver also gets 32 percent of its calories from fat, and contains 530 mg of cholesterol per 3-ounce serving.

Duck: Americans eat less than a pound of duck per person, per year. Duck is a fatty meat, with about 50 percent of its calories coming from fat. Three ounces of roasted duck supply 20 to 25 percent of the RDA for riboflavin (B_2), iron and niacin, plus smaller amounts of thiamin (B_1), B_6, B_{12}, potassium, and zinc.

Goose: Goose is generally higher in calories and fat than turkey, getting 45 to 50 percent of its calories from fat. A 3-ounce serving of roasted goose meat supplies a good amount of protein and 20 to 25 percent of the RDA for iron, vitamins B_6 and B_{12}, with smaller amounts of riboflavin (B_1), folic acid, niacin, magnesium, potassium, and zinc.

Including the Food in Your Diet

Three ounces of lean poultry per day is enough to give most people enough protein for good health. (Remember, you also get protein from dairy products, vegetables, and grains.) Thomas Jefferson's approach to meat and poultry is perhaps the best: He used it as a condiment, rather than as the main dish.

CHICKEN BREAST
3 oz roasted, meat only

Calories	142	
Protein	26.7 gm	
Carbohydrate	0 gm	
Fat	3.1 gm	
Cholesterol	73 mg	
Dietary Fiber	0 gm	

	Amount	RDA
Niacin	11.8 mg	59%
Vitamin B_6	0.5	25%

CHICKEN DRUMSTICKS
1, meat only (approx. 0.5 oz)

Calories	76	
Protein	12.4 gm	
Carbohydrate	0 gm	
Fat	2.5 gm	
Cholesterol	41 mg	
Dietary Fiber	0 gm	

	Amount	RDA
Niacin	2.7 mg	14%
Vitamin B_6	0.2 mg	10%

TURKEY
dark meat, roasted, 5 oz

Calories	262	
Protein	40 gm	
Carbohydrate	0 gm	
Fat	10.1 gm	
Cholesterol	119 mg	
Dietary Fiber	0 gm	

	Amount	RDA
Zinc	6.3 mg	42%
Niacin	5.1 mg	26%
Vitamin B_6	0.5 mg	25%
Phosphorus	169 mg	14%

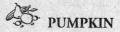

PUMPKIN

No one is quite sure where or when the first pumpkin developed, although we know that even in Colonial times, people were trying to grow giant jack-o'-lanterns. A Connecticut settler named Joshua Hempsted described a pumpkin just shy of six feet in circumference in a diary entry dated 1721. As they did with watermelon, the Colonists fermented pumpkin (with persimmons and sugar) to make beer. They also drank ground pumpkin seeds mixed with water to cure bladder and "female" diseases.

The Pumpkin's Healing Properties

A ½ cup serving of pumpkin provides over 250 percent of the RDA for beta-carotene, plus 11 percent of the iron, 9 percent of the C, and a good amount of fiber.

Beta-carotene is one of 400 carotenes found in foods. Beta-carotene is a "provitamin A" which has vitamin A–like activities in the body, and can be converted into vitamin A by the body as necessary. Among their many effects in the body, beta-carotene and other carotenes help to prevent the transformation of normal cells into cancerous ones. Many studies have found that a low intake of vegetables and fruits containing carotenoids, especially beta-carotene, is strongly associated with an increased risk of lung cancer. Many other cancers, including cancers of the cervix, colon, esophagus, stomach, and skin have also been related to low intakes of foods containing beta and other carotenes.

Pumpkin's fiber also protects against many types of cancer, including cancers of the colon, rectum, prostate, and breast. And people eating high-fiber diets are much less likely to develop constipation or hemorrhoids.

Including the Food in Your Diet

Low in calories and loaded with beta-carotene, cooked pumpkin can be eaten as a side vegetable, much like squash.

It can also be added to a variety of foods, such as soup, bread, muffins, pancakes, and pie. A delicious pumpkin custard can be made from pumpkin, milk, sweetener, and spices.

PUMPKIN ½ cup, canned		
Calories	41	
Protein	1.3 gm	
Carbohydrate	9.9 gm	
Fat	0.3 gm	
Cholesterol	0 mg	
Dietary Fiber	3.4 gm	
	Amount	RDA
Vitamin A	2691 RE	269%
Iron	1.7 mg	11%
Vitamin C	5.1 mg	9%
Folacin	15 mcg	8%
Magnesium	28 mg	7%
Potassium	251 mg	NA

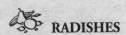 **RADISHES**

Believed to have originated in western Asia, the radish was held in high esteem in the ancient world. The Egyptians even painted radishes on the walls of their tombs. The Greeks carried the vegetable on plates of gold as they marched it into the temples to be burned as an offering to the gods. The less-respectful Romans tossed radishes at speakers they thought were rattling on too long.

In times past radishes had been used as an antidote to poison and snake bites, to relieve the pain of childbirth, to take freckles off the face, and to put hair back on the head.

The Radish's Healing Properties

Although the radish is not a nutritional standout, it does contain a good amount of vitamin C, as well as folic acid, fiber, and other nutrients. And, as a member of the crucifer family of vegetables, it helps to fight cancer. Crucifers contain substances called indoles that can "turn off" the estrogen hormones that may spur the growth of breast and other tumors. The folic acid in radishes also helps to control cancer by strengthening the immune system.

Including the Food in Your Diet

Very low in fat, crispy, and with a "sharp" taste, radishes are a tasty and healthful addition to most any meal or snack. Thinly sliced radishes liven up salad. They're also great as a "finger food" along with sliced carrots, celery, and broccoli pieces. If you dip your radishes, be sure to use a low-fat dip, such as yogurt and herbs, or a nonfat salad dressing.

RADISHES
½ cup sliced, raw

Calories	10	
Protein	0.4 gm	
Carbohydrate	2.0 gm	
Fat	0.3 gm	
Cholesterol	0 mg	
Dietary Fiber	1.3 mg	

	Amount	RDA
Vitamin C	13.2 mg	22%
Folacin	15.7 mcg	8%

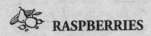 **RASPBERRIES**

Delicate and hollow, raspberries have a relatively brief shelf life. Most raspberries sold in the market are red, but the fruit also ocomes in purple, yellow, amber, and other colors.

The Raspberry's Healing Properties

The vitamin C and folic acid in raspberries help to control oxidative damage to body cells, strengthen the immune system, and stave off the appearance of the signs of aging. The excellent amounts of vitamin C in raspberries help the body absorb the fruit's iron, meaning that more of the fruit's iron is "bioavailable," and can actually be used by the body.

With large amounts of fiber, raspberries help to relieve constipation and to reduce the risk of cancer of the colon, rectum, pancreas, prostate, and breast.

In addition, raspberries contain natural aspirin-like substances. Future studies may show us how to use raspberries in pain prevention and treatment programs.

Including the Food in Your Diet

Low in fat and calories, with absolutely no cholesterol, raspberries make an excellent snack or addition to a fruit salad. Enjoy them often when they are in season, counting them as part of the five or more daily servings of fruits and vegetables recommended by the Food & Nutrition Board.

RASPBERRIES
1 cup, raw

	Amount	
Calories	61	
Protein	1.2 gm	
Carbohydrate	14.3 gm	
Fat	0.7 gm	
Cholesterol	0 mg	
Dietary Fiber	5.8 gm	

	Amount	RDA
Vitamin C	30.8 mg	51%
Folacin	32 mcg	16%
Magnesium	22 mg	6%
Iron	0.7 mg	5%

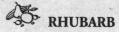 **RHUBARB**

Native to Russia, rhubarb was prized for its laxative properties in Asia 3,000 years before Christ. The English name for the vegetable comes from the Greeks, who referred to it, in a rather unfriendly manner, as "the plant eaten by those barbarians living on the other side of the river."

Rhubarb was brought to the United States in the latter half of the 1700s, where it was used in pies and preserves for many years. Unfortunately, the hapless vegetable came under a cloud of suspicion during World War I, and was accused of poisoning people who ate it. (The real culprit turned out to be the rhubarb leaf, rather than the stalks which are normally eaten.)

Rhubarb's Healing Properties

Unfortunately, rhubarb's ancient laxative properties have been bred out of today's supermarket version of the vegetable. However, the modern rhubarb does contain fiber, vitamin C, potassium, and other nutrients. Rhubarb also contains calcium, but it is in the form of calcium oxalate, which the body has difficulty absorbing.

Including the Food in Your Diet

Rhubarb can be baked, boiled in a sugar water solution, used in salad molds, cobblers, and pies, or made into preserves. When the tart vegetable is mixed in a sweet sauce, the combination of tart and sweet is delicious. Usually prepared as a side dish, rhubarb should be eaten several times a week.

Caution: The oxalate in rhubarb may encourage the formation of kidney stones. People with a personal or family history of stones may want to consider restricting or avoiding rhubarb and other high-oxalate foods, such as spinach and swiss chard.

RHUBARB
½ cup raw, diced

Calories	13
Protein	0.5 gm
Carbohydrate	2.8 gm
Fat	0.1 gm
Cholesterol	0 mg
Dietary Fiber	1.1 gm

	Amount	RDA
Vitamin C	5.0 mg	8%
Calcium	52 mg	4%
Potassium	175 mg	NA

RICE

Native to India, rice is a dietary staple in many countries. In fact, the word for "eat" in some languages literally means "eat rice." Although no one can trace the movement of the grain with certainty, rice may have been brought to the Western world by Alexander the Great in the fourth century B.C.

Ancient Eastern cultures associated rice with fertility. Here in the United States we do the same, throwing rice at newlywed couples. In addition, throughout history, rice has been used to treat diarrhea, high blood pressure, and urinary problems.

Brown Rice's Healing Properties

Low in fat, brown rice contains excellent amounts of thiamin (vitamin B_1), plus magnesium, vitamin B_6, niacin, iron, and fiber.

Just ½ cup of cooked brown rice provides 67 percent of the RDA for thiamin, the first of the B-vitamins to be discovered. Thiamin helps to ensure that all the body cells, especially nerve cells, run smoothly. A lack of thiamin is felt to allow metabolic "trash" to pile up within the cells, hampering their efficiency and leading to a variety of nonspecific problems such as weakness, depression, constipation, heightened sensitivity to pain, confusion, and problems with the heart. At least one study has found that low intakes of thiamin are associated with an increased risk of getting prostate cancer.

Within its oil, rice contains natural antioxidants such as ferulic, and all the various members of the natural vitamin E family. These antioxidants and other substances in the rice oil and bran help to control cholesterol levels, while protecting against the cancer-causing effects of unregulated oxidation within the body.

The bran in brown rice contains gamma-oryzanol, a substance which helps to lower cholesterol. Rice also contains protease inhibitors, substances which put a damper on the proteases that encourage the growth of cancer in the body.

White rice is slightly higher in calories than brown rice, and has less dietary fiber. It loses nutrients during the processing, some of which are later added back. All in all, brown rice is more nutritious, and just as tasty, as white rice.

Including the Food in Your Diet

Brown rice should be a frequent visitor to your dinner table. The Food & Nutrition Board recommends eating six or more servings per day of foods high in complex carbohydrates, such as brown rice, beans, and peas. A serving or more per day of rice will help to keep your cholesterol under control, and help you meet that dietary goal.

RICE, WHITE, ENRICHED
½ cup, cooked

Calories	133
Protein	2.4 gm
Carbohydrate	29.2 gm
Fat	0.2 gm
Cholesterol	0 mg
Dietary Fiber	0.2 gm

	Amount	RDA
Thiamin	0.2 mg	13%
Iron	1.5 mg	10%
Niacin	1.9 mg	10%

RICE, BROWN
½ **cup, cooked**

Calories	110	
Protein	2.3 gm	
Carbohydrate	230 gm	
Fat	0.8 gm	
Cholesterol	0 mg	
Dietary Fiber	1.7 gm	

	Amount	RDA
Thiamin	1.0 mg	67%
Magnesium	43 mg	11%
Vitamin B$_6$	0.2 mg	10%
Niacin	1.0 mg	5%
Iron	0.5 mg	3%

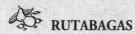 **RUTABAGAS**

Sometimes called "Swedes" because they are popular in Sweden, the rutabaga was developed in the 1700s by a European botanist who wanted to see what would happen when turnips and cabbages were cross-bred.

The Rutabaga's Healing Properties

A member of the crucifer family of vegetables, the rutabaga contains indoles and other substances which help to prevent the formation and spread of various types of cancer. Rutabagas also contain excellent amounts of folic acid, very good levels of vitamin C, plus potassium, magnesium, fiber, and other nutrients.

The folic acid in rutabagas may be of special value in preventing cancer of the cervix. Since women using birth control pills are vulnerable to cervical cancer, researchers looked at 47 such women who already had mild to moderate alterations in cervical cells. Some of the women were given folic acid, the others a placebo. Three months later, a new sampling of cervical cells from the women who had received the folic acid looked much healthier than did cells from the placebo group.

The rutabaga's potassium helps to keep blood pressure at healthy levels, and the heart beating properly, while the vegetable's vitamin C strengthens the immune system and fights off the dangerous oxidants that can damage body cells.

Including the Food in Your Diet

Rutabagas are commonly baked like potatoes and served mashed, or added to mashed potatoes. Low in fat, these cancer-fighting crucifers should be a regular addition to your diet.

RUTABAGAS
½ cup cubes, baked

Calories	30
Protein	0.9 gm
Carbohydrate	8.2 gm
Fat	0.1 gm
Cholesterol	0 mg
Dietary Fiber	1.1 mg

	Amount	RDA
Vitamin C	18.6 mg	31%
Folacin	132 mcg	7%
Potassium	244 mg	NA

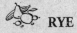 RYE

Native to Asia, rye is a close relative of wheat. Although rye was eaten as a breakfast cereal in Colonial America, today it is much more likely to find its way into rye whiskey and other alcoholic beverages, or in breads.

Rye's Healing Properties

Although rye does not have outstanding amounts of any single nutrient, it is a nutritional cornucopia containing phosphorus, magnesium, iron, folic acid, zinc, riboflavin, vitamin B_6, vitamin E, copper, manganese, and dietary fiber. Rye bread and other rye products may help dieters lose weight. Rye fiber contains substances called noncellulose polysaccharides, which attach themselves to water in the intestines, giving you a feeling of fullness and helping to cut back on the appetite.

Including the Food in Your Diet

Breads made from all rye flour tend to be heavy, dense, and flat (like pumpernickel). The typical loaf of rye bread on the market is not all rye. Instead, it contains a great deal of wheat flour, and less rye than you might think. Some rye bread has sourdough added for flavor.

In baking, a cup of rye meal (whole rye flour, coarsely ground) can stand in for a cup of all-purpose flour. Whole rye berries look like wheat berries and can be cooked like rice. Cracked rye, which is also prepared like rice, cooks up more quickly than does whole rye. Rye flakes look like oatmeal, and may be cooked and eaten as if they were.

RYE
½ cup, raw

Calories	280	
Protein	12.4 gm	
Carbohydrate	58.5 gm	
Fat	2.2 gm	
Cholesterol	0 mg	
Dietary Fiber	—	

	Amount	RDA
Folacin	50.4 mcg	25%
Iron	2.2 mg	15%
Magnesium	52 mg	13%

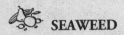 **SEAWEED**

Often called kelp, seaweed is actually a group of plant foods that come from the sea. Kelp, nori, sea lettuce, and Irish moss are all forms of seaweed. In Egypt and Asia, seaweed has long been used to treat cancer. In various places and at various times, it has also been used to assuage arthritis, skin diseases, ulcers, obesity, and urinary problems.

Seaweed's Healing Properties

Seaweed also contains good amounts of folacin, plus magnesium, calcium, potassium, iodine, iron, and fiber. Various studies suggest that seaweed may help to:

- Fight cancer
- Slow the development of herpes

Seaweed may also strengthen the immune system, thin the blood, reduce blood pressure, and help in treating ulcers.

What Scientists Have Learned About Seaweed

Seaweed and Cancer: A Harvard researcher who knew that the Japanese have much less cancer than do Americans wondered if seaweed might have some anticancer properties. After all, the Japanese ate a lot of seaweed but had relatively little cancer, while Americans ate practically no seaweed, but were much more prone to developing the terrible disease.

Studies with laboratory animals showed that substances in various types of seaweed not only helped to prevent the onset of breast and other cancers, but also slowed the rate at which these cancers spread, if they were already present. The anticancer ingredient in seaweed was later identified as fuciodan.

Seaweed and Herpes: Herpes Simplex I and II have become major health concerns since the 1980s. (Herpes I causes cold sores, while Herpes II produces genital herpes.) Substances in seaweed have demonstrated anti-herpes properties in the laboratory at the University of California at Berkeley. There, human cells which contained the viruses were mixed with various types of seaweed extract. The seaweed was able to slow the progress of the virus, cutting back on its ability to spread itself by about half. When human cells were pretreated with seaweed extract before being exposed to the herpes virus, the anti-herpes effect was even stronger.

Including the Food in Your Diet

Crushed seaweed is a tasty addition to many soups, and rolling boiled rice in seaweed turns the grain into a ''finger food.'' Let your creativity be your only limit to how much seaweed you add to your diet.

SEAWEED (KELP)
1 oz, raw

Calories	12	
Protein	0.5 gm	
Carbohydrate	2.6 gm	
Fat	0.2 gm	
Cholesterol	0 mg	
Dietary Fiber	0.1 gm	

	Amount		RDA
Folacin	50	mcg	25%
Magnesium	34	mg	9%

 SEEDS

From the prehistoric past right up to the present day, seeds have been the single most important food category. Grains, nuts, peas, beans, and lentils are all seeds: compact sources of protein, carbohydrate, and/or fat, that are easy to transport and simple to store. Today, well over 60 percent of the protein consumed by humans the world over comes from seeds.

Although good sources of protein, seeds provide incomplete protein, missing one or more of the amino acids that make up protein. (Which amino acids are missing depend on the seed.) That's why various cultures around the world have learned to combine seed foods to make complete proteins. For example, both beans and corn contain incomplete proteins. But since they are missing different amino acids, and each has what the other lacks, a diet which includes beans plus corn or rice is a good source of complete protein. Indeed, the traditional Central American diet is based on those two foods.

Since grains, peas, beans, and lentils have been discussed elsewhere, this section looks at sunflower seeds, pumpkin seeds and sesame seeds (the things we normally think of when seeds are mentioned).

Seeds' Healing Properties

Seeds contain a variety of nutrients, including vitamin E, iron, potassium, protein, and fiber. Sunflower seeds contain linoleic acid, an essential fatty acid that has shown promise in reducing the risk of heart disease by controlling cholesterol. Pumpkin seeds, which contain essential fatty acids and zinc, have been used to treat prostate enlargement and intestinal parasites. Sesame seeds contain *sesamin,* an antioxidant which counteracts the dangerous oxidation reactions within the body that can encourage cancer, heart disease and a host of other problems. Sesamin may also help to lower total cholesterol.

Thanks to their protease inhibitors, seeds help to slow the growth of cancer by interfering with the proteases that encourage cancers to grow. Protease inhibitors also have antioxidant properties. Like vitamins A, C, and E, protease inhibitors also serve as antioxidants.

Including the Food in Your Diet

Seeds have health-enhancing properties. Use seeds as an occasional delicious substitute for small amounts of meat, cheese, or other fatty foods. You can also add small amounts of seeds to salads, vegetable and pasta dishes.

SUNFLOWER SEEDS
1 oz, dried

Calories	162
Protein	6.5 gm
Carbohydrate	5.3 gm
Fat	14.1 gm
Cholesterol	0 mg
Dietary Fiber	1.3 gm

	Amount	RDA
Thiamin	0.6 mg	40%
Folacin	64.6 mcg	32%
Magnesium	100 mg	25%
Iron	1.9 mg	13%
Vitamin B$_6$	0.2 mg	10%
Zinc	1.4 mg	9%
Niacin	1.3 mg	7%
Potassium	196 mg	NA

PUMPKIN SEEDS
1 oz dried, hulled

Calories	154
Protein	7.0 gm
Carbohydrate	5.1 gm
Fat	13.0 gm
Cholesterol	0 mg
Dietary Fiber	3.9 gm

	Amount	RDA
Magnesium	151.9 mg	38%
Iron	4.3 mg	29%
Zinc	2.1 mg	14%
Folacin	16.3 mcg	8%
Riboflavin	0.1 mg	6%
Potassium	229 mg	NA

SOY (Including Soybeans, Tofu, Miso, and Tempeh)

Soy beans, which are legumes, are related to other beans, peas, and lentils. Long a staple in Asia, soybeans can be eaten cooked or sprouted, or turned into tofu, miso, tempeh, soy milk, soy sauce, and soy flour.

Native to northern China and used throughout Asia for centuries, the soybean was brought back to the United States by Commodore Matthew Perry, who visited Japan in 1854. Although immediately planted by American farmers, it was not used in foods because the unstable oil in soy is likely to develop a funny taste or go rancid quickly. Instead, soybeans were grown and their oil used to make soap and paint. Soybeans did not become a major food crop until the mid-1900s, when a process called hydrogenation made it possible to stabilize soy oil, keeping it fresh and making it useful in foods such as margarine.

We eat soy in many forms. One of these, tofu, is curdled soy milk. An excellent source of protein, tofu also contains good amounts of iron, magnesium and calcium, plus zinc and fiber. Be on guard, however, for tofu is surprisingly high in fat. Soy is also mixed with either wheat or barley and made into a fermented mix called miso, or combined with grains and culture to produce tempeh.

Soy's Healing Properties

Serious scientific studies, many of them conducted in Japan, have identified several health benefits enjoyed by people who eat soybeans and soy products. Soy may help to:

• Reduce the risk of cancer
• Moderate the symptoms of menopause
• Keep the bones and memory strong

What Scientists Have Learned About Soy

Soy and Cancer: According to a report published in the National Cancer Institute's journal, "Soy products lower the risk of several forms of cancer, over and above their low-fat, high-fiber content. They contain several anti-cancer compounds, including phytoestrogens such as isoflavones, protease inhibitors, phytosterols and saponins."

Isoflavones interfere with estrogen's ability to interact with and encourage the growth of certain tumor cells. Protease inhibitors slow or halt the growth of cancers of the colon, lungs, liver, pancreas, and esophagus. Saponins kill cancer cells directly and indirectly by strengthening the immune system's natural fighting abilities. These powerful substances can slow the growth of cancers of the colon, cervix, and skin. Soybeans also help to disarm nitrosamines, powerful carcinogens which can cause liver and other cancers. In addition, the folic acid in soy helps to protect against cervical and possibly lung cancer.

Soy has demonstrated quite an ability to protect against stomach cancer. Researchers in Japan have found that eating a single bowl of miso soup every day reduces the risk of stomach cancer by two-thirds.

Soy and Menopause: Japanese women, who eat much more tofu and other soy products than do American women, tend to have much less discomfort when they move into menopause. This may largely be because soybeans and soybean products contain isoflavones, which act as "almost estrogens," mimicking the effects of natural estrogen and relieving many of the discomforting symptoms of menopause. A recent Australian study found that eating 45 grams of soy flour every day for about three months cut the number of hot flashes in menopausal women by 40 percent (without the side effects suffered by many women on hormone replacement therapy).

Including the Food in Your Diet

Adding tofu to stir-fries or soups, enjoying a frequent bowl of miso soup, or using soybeans in place of other beans in recipes will strengthen your resistance to cancer and other ailments.

SOYBEAN SPROUTS
½ cup, raw

Calories	45	
Protein	4.6 gm	
Carbohydrate	3.9 gm	
Fat	2.4 gm	
Cholesterol	0 mg	
Dietary Fiber	—	

	Amount	RDA
Folacin	60.1 mcg	30%
Vitamin C	5.4 mg	9%

TOFU
¼ block (approx. 4 oz)

Calories	90	
Protein	9.4 gm	
Carbohydrate	2.2 gm	
Fat	5.4 gm	
Cholesterol	0 mg	
Dietary Fiber	1.4 gm	

	Amount	RDA
Iron	6.2 mg	41%
Magnesium	120 mg	30%
Calcium	122 mg	10%

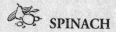 SPINACH

Native to Asia, spinach was brought to Europe by the Moors when they conquered Spain in the eighth century A.D. Although medieval monks were limited to spinach and a few other foods on fast days, the French King Louis XIV was furious when his doctors told him that he could not eat the leafy green vegetable he enjoyed so much. Furious, he yelled: "I am the king of France and I cannot eat spinach!" He got his spinach.

An article published in *American Medicine* in 1927 was just as favorably inclined toward spinach. The authors of the article suggested that spinach should be used to treat heart and kidney problems, anemia, "low vitality and marked general debility."

Spinach's Healing Properties

Although eating spinach will not cause one to develop instant muscles, à la Popeye, the vegetable goes a long way toward building good health. Studies suggest that spinach may:

- guard against cancer
- reduce the risk of heart disease
- protect the vision
- help to stave off depression

What Scientists Have Learned About Spinach

Spinach and Cancer: Spinach is also one of the best sources of a class of phytochemicals called carotenoids—the best known of which is beta-carotene. Spinach also has large amounts of chlorophyll (which gives the vegetable its green color), believed by some researchers to block initiation, the first step in the transformation of normal cells to cancerous killers.

Large-scale population studies have found that people who eat more dark, leafy vegetables, such as spinach, have fewer cancers of the lung, cervix, prostate, stomach, colon, rectum, esophagus, and endometrium. The studies have shown that even former smokers can significantly reduce the risk of lung cancer by eating spinach, or other carotene-containing vegetables, every day.

Spinach and the Heart: Back in 1969, Japanese researchers noted that giving spinach to laboratory animals lowered their cholesterol levels. More recent studies have shown that spinach encourages the transformation of excess cholesterol to coprostanol, which the body washes away.

Spinach and Vision: Studies have shown that people eating larger amounts of spinach have a lower risk of cataracts, a condition resulting from a clouding of the normally clear lens of the eye. A Harvard Medical School study found that spinach is actually better at protecting against cataracts than are carrots, even though carrots are great sources of beta-carotene. The vision-heroes in spinach may be the lutein and zeaxanthin which are found in high amounts in spinach (but in lower amounts in carrots).

Spinach and Mood: Spinach contains excellent amounts of the B-vitamin called folacin (folic acid). A deficiency of folacin has been associated with forgetfulness, irritability, and sleeplessness, as well as with depression, schizophrenia, and dementia. In a fascinating study, 200 mcg of folic acid were given daily to 75 depressed, medicated patients. This dose of folic acid, equivalent to the amount found in less than a cup of cooked spinach, significantly relieved the patients' depression.

Including the Food in Your Diet

Eating spinach several times a week, whether steamed as a side dish or raw in salads, or sautéed with a bit of olive oil and garlic, adds a great deal of tasty nutrition to the diet. The nutrients and phytochemicals in spinach will help to keep your cholesterol under control, cancer at bay, and your vision sharp.

But do not rely on spinach as an important dietary source of iron or calcium. The body cannot utilize most of the iron and calcium in spinach, for both of these minerals tend to bind with other substances in the vegetable, making them difficult for the body to absorb.

> **Caution:** *Spinach is not recommended for those with kidney stones, or a tendency toward them, for it may contribute to the making of the stones.*

SPINACH
½ cup, cooked

Calories	21
Protein	2.7 gm
Carbohydrate	3.4 gm
Fat	0.2 gm
Cholesterol	0 mg
Dietary Fiber	1.7 gm

	Amount	RDA
Vitamin A	737 RE	74%
Folacin	131.2 mcg	66%
Iron	3.2 mg	21%
Magnesium	78.3 mg	20%
Calcium	122.4 mg	10%

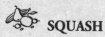 **SQUASH**

Native to the Americas, squash was cultivated perhaps as long as 9,000 years ago in Mexico. Native Americans ate squash seeds to expel worms, and used squash juice to treat snakebites. Colonial Americans used squash paste for black eyes and toothaches, and "squash-water" or whole squash to cure bladder ailments and to relieve the pain of childbirth.

Squash's Healing Properties

Although each type of squash has a unique nutritional profile, in general the various squashes contain beta-carotene, vitamin C, B-vitamins, and fiber. Low in fat and very high in water, the fiber-containing vegetables are low-calorie additions to the diet.

Including the Food in Your Diet

Eating the mild-tasting squash is a nutritious way to bolster your immune system and improve your general health without adding too many calories to the diet. Eat it several times a week, steamed, baked, or grated into salads.

ACORN SQUASH
½ cup cubes, baked

Calories	57
Protein	1.1 gm
Carbohydrate	14.9 gm
Fat	0.1 gm
Cholesterol	0 mg
Dietary Fiber	2.9 gm

	Amount	RDA
Vitamin C	11 mg	18%
Thiamin	0.2 mg	13%
Magnesium	44 mg	11%
Potassium	445.7 mg	NA

SPAGHETTI SQUASH
½ cup cubes, baked

Calories	51	
Protein	3.0 gm	
Carbohydrate	11.0 gm	
Fat	0.6 gm	
Cholesterol	0 mg	
Dietary Fiber	2.9 gm	

	Amount		RDA
Vitamin A	616	RE	62%
Vitamin C	10	mg	17%
Potassium	365	mg	NA

ZUCCHINI SQUASH
½ cup cubes, baked

Calories	14	
Protein	0.6 gm	
Carbohydrate	3.5 gm	
Fat	0.1 gm	
Cholesterol	0 mg	
Dietary Fiber	1.3 gm	

	Amount	RDA
Folacin	15.1 mcg	8%
Vitamin C	4.1 mg	7%

STRAWBERRIES

The most popular of all berries, the strawberry is native to the Americas as well as to Europe. Ancient Romans, the Medieval French, and American Indians grew and ate the berry. The seventy-some varieties of our modern strawberry are descended from a large-berried version brought from Chili to Europe some 300 years ago by a French engineer.

Throughout history, strawberry juices and preparations have been used to treat various types of skin problems, fevers, and gum problems.

The Strawberry's Healing Properties

Low in fat and calories, strawberries are overflowing with vitamin C, with one cup of raw berries offering just over 140 percent of the RDA for C. Strawberries also contain fiber, folic acid, potassium, iron, and riboflavin. And in laboratory experiments, strawberry extract has destroyed a variety of viruses, including herpes simplex.

Strawberries contains *p*-coumaric acid and chloregenic acid, two little-known substances which help reduce the risk of cancer by "sticking to" the nitric oxides from our food. "Gummed up" by the *p*-coumaric acid and chloregenic acid, the nitric oxides are flushed out of the body before they can be transformed into the nitrosamines, which raise the risk of cancer.

The vitamin C in strawberries helps the T-cells, B-cells, and other components of the immune system attack and destroy foreign invaders and cancerous growths within the body. And, as an antioxidant, vitamin C helps to prevent the damage to cellular DNA that might turn normal cells cancerous. The vitamin is assisted in the fight against cancer by strawberry's ellagic acid, which disarms certain cancer-causing substances before they have an opportunity to act, as well as by the fruit's fiber, which guards against cancers of the colon, rectum, pancreas, breast, and prostate.

The tremendous amounts of C in strawberries may explain

why the berry has long been used as a home remedy for skin problems. During a study at the University of California at San Francisco, 10 people with severe eczema, a disease that makes the skin thick, crusted, and scaly, were given vitamin C for a period of time, then a placebo for the same amount of time. The volunteers, ranging in age from 3 to 21, noted a decrease in symptoms and required half as much medication while taking the vitamin.

Dieters, take note: At least one study has shown that taking 3 grams of supplemental vitamin C can help the obese to lose weight.

Including the Food in Your Diet

When they are in season, several weekly servings of strawberries will help to keep you healthy, from your skin all the way to your heart. Fresh strawberries are delicious by themselves; they don't need to be covered with high-fat cream or with sugar.

STRAWBERRIES
1 cup, raw

Calories	45	
Protein	1.0 gm	
Carbohydrate	10.5 gm	
Fat	0.6 gm	
Cholesterol	0 mg	
Dietary Fiber	2.9 gm	

	Amount	RDA
Vitamin C	84.5 mg	141%
Folacin	26.4 mg	13%
Iron	0.6 mg	4%
Potassium	247 mg	NA

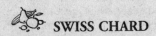 **SWISS CHARD**

Swiss chard is the green, leafy part of a type of beet grown specifically for its leafy top, rather than its root. In one form or another, chard has been eaten for thousands of years in Asia Minor, the Middle East, Greece, and Rome. The Greek philosopher Aristotle mentioned chard in his writings hundreds of years before the Common Era.

Swiss Chard's Healing Properties

This green, leafy vegetable is a very good source of beta-carotene and vitamin C. It also offers magnesium, iron, potassium, and calcium. Beta-carotene and vitamin C help the immune system fight off viruses, cancers, and other challenges. They also slow the oxidation of the LDL (''bad'') cholesterol. This helps the heart, for LDL is more likely to leave deposits on the artery walls when it has been oxidized. Magnesium helps to keep the heart beating regularly, also reduces the total cholesterol and LDL in some people, and can increase the survival rate of heart attack victims.

Including the Food in Your Diet

A delightful but overlooked green, Swiss chard can regularly be added to salads, either chopped or as whole leaves. Or it can be steamed or sautéed in margarine or olive oil. With its beta-carotene, vitamin C, magnesium, and iron, it is a healthful addition to any diet.

> *Caution: Swiss chard contains a large amount of oxalates, substances which may encourage the formation of kidney stones. People with a personal or family history of stones may want to consider restricting or avoiding high-oxalate foods such as Swiss chard, rhubarb, and spinach.*

SWISS CHARD
½ cup chopped, cooked

Calories	18	
Protein	1.6 gm	
Carbohydrate	3.6 gm	
Fat	0.1 gm	
Cholesterol	0 mg	
Dietary Fiber	1.8 gm	

	Amount	RDA
Vitamin A	276 RE	28%
Vitamin C	15.8 mg	26%
Magnesium	76 mg	19%
Iron	2.0 mg	13%
Potassium	483 mg	NA

 TANGERINES

Although often referred to as "mandarins," the tangerine, like the tangelo, the Clementine, and the Temple, is just one of the many varieties of the mandarin orange. The small orange fruit, which has been grown and eaten in Asia for more than 4,000 years, is said to have been named for the city of Tangier, Morocco. The tangerine was brought from Italy to Louisiana by the Italian Counsel in the mid-1800s.

The Tangerine's Healing Properties

Like its cousin the orange, the tangerine contains vitamin C, beta-carotene, folic acid and pectin fiber. Vitamin C helps to strengthen the immune system, ward off cancer, and lessen the risk of heart disease. Beta-carotene protects the heart and strengthens the body's resistance to cancer. Folic acid helps to keep the immune system strong and aids in proper growth. Pectin, a soluble fiber found in the tangerine's membranes and skin, protects against heart disease by lowering the total cholesterol and LDL cholesterol, while raising HDL cholesterol.

Including the Food in Your Diet

The Food & Nutrition Board recommends eating five or more servings of fruits and vegetables per day. With plenty of nutrients and lots of good taste, tangerines should be a regular part of that allotment when they are in season.

TANGERINES
1 raw (approx. 3 oz)

Calories	37	
Protein	0.6 gm	
Carbohydrate	9.4 gm	
Fat	0.2 gm	
Cholesterol	0 mg	
Dietary Fiber	—	

	Amount	RDA
Folacin	17.1 mcg	9%
Vitamin A	77 RE	8%
Vitamin C	2.6 mg	4%

TEAS

The Ancient Chinese, the Greeks, Medieval herbalists, scholars of the Enlightenment, and physicians right up to the modern era have found many medicinal uses for tea. Black or green, standard or exotic, tea has been used to treat colds, asthma, headaches, heart disease, elevated blood pressure, and many other common ailments.

Black tea, green tea, and oolong tea are derived from the *Camellia sinensis* plant. Herbal teas, which are made up of herbs and spices, may not contain any actual tea at all. Instead they are made from the flowers, stems, and roots of various plants.

Tea's Healing Properties

Black tea, green tea, and oolong tea have been put to the test in many laboratory and epidemiological studies. The evidence suggests that tea may help to:

• Keep the arteries healthy
• Prevent heart disease and stroke
• Fight cancer
• Fight off infections

The caffeine in tea also acts as an analgesic to reduce pain, and a diuretic to help flush excess water out of the body.

What Scientists Have Learned About Tea

Tea and the Heart: Medical researchers have long been intrigued by the fact that the Japanese and Chinese suffer from far less heart disease than do Americans. Indeed, autopsies of soldiers killed in battle during the Korean War showed that while the young American men had the beginnings of blockages in their coronary arteries, the young Koreans did not.

One obvious avenue of research was to compare the low-fat Asian diet to the high-fat American diet. Another was to look at the individual foods or drinks that were much more popular in Asia than in the United States—such as tea.

If you feed laboratory animals a high-fat, high-cholesterol diet, their arteries will eventually become blocked, and they will develop heart disease. If you give them the same diet *plus* either black or green tea, their arteries will suffer less damage. Tea undoubtedly has the same positive effects in humans, for the heart and brain arteries of Chinese-Americans who regularly drink tea have much less damage than do the same arteries in Americans who prefer coffee. We now know that tannins and possibly other substances in tea help to keep arteries healthy by keeping the blood "thin." Thin blood is less likely to form unnecessary clots which can stick to the artery walls and cause blockages.

Tea and Cancer: Black, green, and oolong tea contain anti-cancer fighting substances called catechins. These and possibly other substances in tea significantly retard the development of skin, stomach, and lung cancer in mice. Even mice who were exposed to cigarette smoke developed much less cancer when their drinking water was mixed with compounds taken from tea.

Tea and Infections: The tannins in tea act as antiviral and antibacterial agents. Thanks to scientific discoveries dating back to the 1940s, we know that tea can fight herpes simplex, at least one form of influenza (flu), and other viruses. Japanese researchers have reported that green tea can help to keep cavities under control by killing *streptococcus mutans*, the bacteria that promote cavities.

Including the Drink in Your Diet

A glass of green tea every day will help to protect against heart disease and cancer. Although black tea has many medicinal properties, the weight of current scientific evidence suggests that green tea is more healthful.

TEA, BLACK 6 oz		
Calories	2	
Protein	0	gm
Carbohydrate	0.5	gm
Fat	0	gm
Cholesterol	0	mg
Dietary Fiber	0	gm
	Amount	RDA
Folacin	9 mcg	5%

TOMATOES

The modern tomato, which is probably descended from the cherry tomato indigenous to South America, has had a strange history. Spanish explorers who brought the tomato back home to Europe in the 1500s thought that it was poisonous. That reputation persisted, in one form or another, for almost four hundred years. The Pilgrims took a dim view of tomatoes, feeling that eating the strange, round, red things was just about as bad as dancing or playing cards. And in 1893 the United States Supreme Court declared that the tomato was a vegetable, which it is not; it's actually a fruit.

Fortunately, the tomato survived these and other outrages to become the third-most-popular vegetable in the United States. Of course, the tomato shouldn't be anywhere on the "Most Popular Vegetables" list because it's really a fruit, but who can argue with the Supreme Court?

The Tomato's Healing Properties

Although not as nutrient-dense as certain other foods, the tomato provides vitamin C, beta-carotene, folate, iron, and potassium. And because the tomato's iron is accompanied by vitamin C, it has a better chance of being absorbed into the body than does unescorted iron. Tomatoes may help to:

- Reduce the risk of cancer
- Lower the risk of appendicitis

What Scientists Have Learned About the Tomato

Tomatoes and Cancer: Like other fruits, tomatoes began showing up on lists of foods eaten by groups of people who suffered from fewer cancers of the bladder, prostate, lung, and other parts of the body. One study of some 17,000 American and Norwegian men found that eating tomatoes, cabbage, or carrots cut the risk of getting lung cancer. A recent Italian study found that eating seven raw tomatoes per week halved the risk of lung cancer and a precancerous condition of the cervix called CIN (cervical intraepithelial neoplasia).

It's probably not the tomato's beta-carotene alone that's responsible for fighting cancer, as the vegetable/fruit is not a particularly good source of this vitamin. But tomatoes are excellent sources of another member of the carotene family called lycopene. A Johns Hopkins University study of 26,000 people found that those with the lowest levels of lycopene in their blood had five times as much cancer as did those with the highest levels of lycopene. The lycopene in tomatoes may protect women against cervical cancer. Studies conducted at the University of Illinois found that women with the highest levels of lycopene in the blood were much less likely to develop CIN, an inflammation of the cervix that may encourage the development of cancer. (Additional protection for the cervix is found in the tomato's folic acid.)

In addition to lycopene, tomatoes are rich in *p*-coumaric acid and chloregenic acid, two substances which bind to the nitric oxides in our food. Thus bound, the nitric oxides are carried out of the body rather than converted into the nitrosamines which can cause cancer.

Tomatoes and Appendicitis: A study conducted in Wales found that eating good amounts of tomatoes confers protection against appendicitis.

Tomatoes, Iron, and Vitamin C: Iron improves resistance to various diseases by strengthening the immune system. Although a single tomato provides only 5 percent of the RDA of iron for men, and 4 percent for women, the tomato's iron is paired with good amounts of vitamin C. The C "escorts" the iron from the digestive system and into the body, making it more available to the body than would otherwise be the case.

Including the Food in Your Diet

Recent studies have shown that eating one tomato a day confers a great deal of protection from cancer.

TOMATOES
1 red ripe (approx. 4.3 oz)

	Amount	
Calories	24	
Protein	1.1 gm	
Carbohydrate	5.3 gm	
Fat	0.3 gm	
Cholesterol	0 mg	
Dietary Fiber	1.0 gm	

	Amount	RDA
Vitamin C	21.6 mg	36%
Vitamin A	139 RE	14%
Folacin	11.6 mcg	6%
Iron	.8 mg	5%

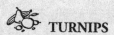 **TURNIPS**

Pity the poor turnip. Although known and eaten since ancient times, it has usually been considered a poor man's food. In fact, English lords put turnips on their coat of arms to indicate that they supported the poor. Despite its humble history, the turnip has been used to treat frostbite, joint aches, the measles and smallpox, and was used to make a beauty soap from Roman times to the Middle Ages.

The Turnip's Healing Properties

Low in fat and calories, the turnip provides fiber and vitamin C. A member of the crucifer family of vegetables, turnips may:

• Aid in the battle against cancer

Turnip greens, the top part of the turnip that is usually thrown away, contain vitamin C and beta-carotene, two antioxidants that protect against cancer and heart disease.

What Scientists Have Learned About the Turnip

Turnips and Cancer: Turnips contain powerful cancer fighters called glucosinolates. Studies at the University of Hawaii have shown that eating large amounts of turnips, turnip greens, and other cruciferous vegetables can significantly reduce the risk of developing lung cancer.

Turnips may also prove to be valuable weapons against breast cancer. The risk of breast cancer is related to the levels of certain forms of estrogen in the body. The indoles in cruciferous vegetables such as turnips speed up the rate at which the body metabolizes estrogens, meaning that there is less estrogen available to promote cancer. The fiber in turnips aids in the fight against cancers of the colon, rectum, pancreas, and prostate.

Including the Food in Your Diet

Making turnips a regular part of your diet will improve your general health while reducing the risk of cancer.

TURNIPS
½ cup cubes, cooked

Calories	14	
Protein	0.6 gm	
Carbohydrate	3.8 gm	
Fat	0.1 gm	
Cholesterol	0 mg	
Dietary Fiber	—	

	Amount	RDA
Vitamin C	9 mg	15%

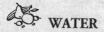 WATER

Water's Healing Properties

Water is essential to health and life. The human body is filled with water: Men's bodies are approximately 60 percent water, while women's bodies are about 50 percent water. In both men and women, the bloodstream, cells, muscles, and brains are watery. Even the bones contain water.

Every day, water is lost via the urine, feces, sweat, and with each exhalation of breath. This water must be replaced if the body is to remain healthy. One can live for three months or more without food, but only 10 to 14 days without water.

Whenever possible, "hard" rather than "soft" water should be the drink of choice. Hard water contains dissolved minerals such as calcium and magnesium, which have a beneficial effect upon health. ("Hardness" may also be caused by the presence of iron or aluminum salts.) People who drink hard water tend to have fewer heart attacks and strokes, and less high blood pressure than those drinking primarily soft water. And the calcium, magnesium, and lithium in hard water may help to protect against cancer of the digestive tract.

Researchers examined the link between hard water and healthy arteries in a study of 27 municipalities in Sweden. In the areas where the water was harder, there were fewer deaths due to heart disease than in the areas where the water was softer. A similar study compared two American cities. In Salt Lake City, where residents get hard water with lots of magnesium from the tap, the death rate from heart attacks is low. But in Washington, D.C., where the tap water is soft and low in magnesium, many more people die of heart attacks.

Water is both an ancient and current treatment for kidney stones. Drinking plenty of water and other fluids helps to keep dissolved calcium and other substances from forming into stones in the kidneys. Instead, the excess substances are swept out of the body with the urine.

Including the Drink in Your Diet

At least eight 8-ounce glasses of water a day are needed to promote good health. Up to twice as much water should be consumed on warm days, or when you are exercising.

Many foods contain what are known as chelating agents that bind up the minerals in the foods, making them difficult or impossible for the body to absorb. Since water generally does not have chelating agents, the minerals in water are often better absorbed than those in certain foods.

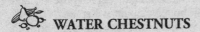 WATER CHESTNUTS

Water chestnuts resemble chestnuts, but they are not nuts. Grown in watery mud, the water chestnut is a white, crunchy vegetable most often seen sliced in Chinese dishes.

The Water Chestnut's Healing Properties

Commonly called the Chinese water chestnut, this sweet, white-fleshed vegetable is low in fat, calories, and sodium, and contains vitamin B_6 and iron. Vitamin B_6 helps the body to turn food into energy. B_6 supplementation has been used to treat certain cases of asthma, premenstrual syndrome, mood and sleep disorders, and carpal tunnel syndrome. Iron improves resistance to various diseases by strengthening the immune system.

Including the Food in Your Diet

Water chestnuts are crunchy and mild-tasting. Add them to your salads and stir-fries, and try them occasionally as a side dish.

WATER CHESTNUTS
canned, ½ cup slices

Calories	35
Protein	0.6 gm
Carbohydrate	8.7 gm
Fat	trace
Cholesterol	0 mg
Dietary Fiber	1.5 mg

	Amount	RDA
Vitamin B_6	0.1 mg	5%
Iron	0.6 mg	4%

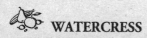 **WATERCRESS**

An often-overlooked member of the crucifer family of vegetables, watercress usually shows up on dinner plates as a garnish. In Brazil, watercress is a native remedy for tuberculosis.

Watercress's Healing Properties

Like cabbage, broccoli, and other members of the cruciferous family of vegetables, watercress contains indoles and other substances which help the body resist cancer. Although watercress itself has not been the subject of many studies, it is well known that people eating diets rich in crucifers, other vegetables, and fresh fruits tend to have lower incidences of various cancers.

Including the Food in Your Diet

Add watercress regularly to your salads. And if you see some watercress acting as garnish on your dinner plate don't just push it to the side—eat it.

WATERCRESS		
½ cup chopped, raw		
Calories	2	
Protein	0.4 gm	
Carbohydrate	0.2 gm	
Fat	trace	
Cholesterol	0 mg	
Dietary Fiber	0.4 gm	
	Amount	RDA
Vitamin C	7.3 mg	12%
Vitamin A	80 RE	8%

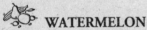 **WATERMELON**

Native to Africa, the watermelon was brought to the United States by early colonists, who sometimes fermented the juice to make melon wine. Watermelon wine was considered a remedy for fevers and other diseases that caused the body to ''heat up.'' But it was for its sweet taste that watermelon was and continues to be prized. As Mark Twain has written, when one has tasted watermelon, ''He knows what the angels eat.''

The Watermelon's Healing Properties

Watermelon contains large concentrations of a red pigment called lycopene. Scientists have only recently learned that lycopene is a powerful antioxidant, perhaps twice as strong as beta-carotene. This makes lycopene—and watermelon—an important weapon in the fight against cancer, heart disease, and the many other ailments associated with oxidation. A study of 26,000 people at Johns Hopkins University found that those with the lowest lycopene levels in the bloodstream were five times more likely to develop cancer of the pancreas as those with the highest levels. Watermelon is a good source of the cancer-fighting antioxidant vitamin C, with one cup of cubes providing 26 percent of the RDA.

In addition to lycopene and vitamin C, watermelon contains beta-carotene, potassium, magnesium, thiamin, and fiber, plus a generous dose of water.

Including the Food in Your Diet

Watermelon is a wonderful summer snack treat and dessert. Eat several slices per week as a delicious source of many vitamins and nutrients, plus phytochemicals such as lycopene.

WATERMELON
1 cup cubes

Calories	51	
Protein	1.0 gm	
Carbohydrate	11.5 gm	
Fat	0.7 gm	
Cholesterol	0 mg	
Dietary Fiber	0.6 gm	

	Amount	RDA
Vitamin C	15.4	26%
Vitamin B$_6$	0.2	10%
Thiamin	0.1 mg	7%
Vitamin A	59 RE	6%
Magnesium	18 mg	5%
Potassium	185 mg	NA

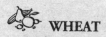 **WHEAT**

The most important cereal crop worldwide, wheat is among the oldest of the cultivated grains. Possibly descended from an Asian strain of grass, wheat was popular in ancient times, lost favor during the Dark and Middle Ages, and reemerged as the preeminent grain during the nineteenth century. Wheat has a long history as a laxative and general health tonic, dating back to the early Greeks.

Today we eat wheat in many forms: wheat berries (groats)—unrefined, untreated kernels of whole wheat; rolled wheat—wheat berries that have been flattened under heavy rollers; cracked wheat—ground-up wheat berries; and bulgur—cracked wheat with additional processing.

Wheat's Healing Properties

Whole-wheat cereal, whole-wheat bread, and wheat bran have many medicinal uses. Wheat may help to:

- Relieve constipation
- Reduce the risk of colon cancer
- Lower the odds of breast cancer in women
- Ward off diverticular disease
- Prevent and treat ulcers

What Scientists Have Learned About Wheat

Wheat and Constipation: Constipation, hemorrhoids, varicose veins, diverticular disease, and other problems related to constipation are a major problem in the Western world, where a highly refined, low-fiber diet is popular. Constipation and its related ailments are rare, however, in parts of the world where people eat a high-fiber diet.

The wheat bran found in wheat is a good source of the insoluble dietary fibers that draw water into the stool as it passes through the intestines, making the stool bulkier. The bulkier stool also moves through the intestines faster, and is easier to eliminate, so straining is not necessary. Many studies conducted at research centers around the world have shown that adding wheat bran, whole-wheat bread, or cereal made from whole wheat to the diet significantly reduces or completely eliminates constipation in up to 70 percent of all sufferers. Since hemorrhoids and varicose veins are sometimes caused by straining, adding good amounts of whole wheat to the diet helps to lessen these problems as well.

Wheat and Cancer: Just as populations eating diets high in whole wheat have less constipation, they also tend to have fewer cancers of the colon and breast. The drop in colon cancer is believed to be due to wheat's ability to make the stool bulkier, diluting the concentration of carcinogens (such as pesticide residues) in the stool. With the carcinogens less likely to come into contact with cells on the walls of the intestines, the risk of cancer is reduced. Something in wheat bran, perhaps its rough texture, may also subtly change the mucus lining the walls of the colon, thereby strengthening the body's defenses against cancer.

Wheat's protective effect against breast cancer is related to a woman's estrogen levels. Wheat bran helps to reduce the elevated levels of certain estrogens that are associated with an elevated risk of breast cancer. (Specifically, wheat fiber reduces the levels of an estrogen called estradiol, which is believed to be associated with breast cancer.) In one study, adding several muffins high in wheat fiber to the daily diet caused estrogen to fall by over 15 percent.

There may be other ways in which wheat helps to protect against cancer. We know, for example, that wheat bran is high in ferulic acid, a compound that has shown anticancer properties in many laboratory studies.

Wheat and Diverticular Disease: Diverticular disease is a "new" problem afflicting up to 40 to 50 percent of those over the age of 60. Diverticular disease (many tiny, inflamed pouches in the lining of the digestive tract) seems to strike primarily those who are eating low-fiber diets. In its most serious form, diverticular disease can cause inflammation of the colon, terrible pain in the lower abdomen, diarrhea, constipation, and cramping.

Doctors insisted that patients with diverticular disease eat only bland foods until a 1972 study in the *British Medical Journal* announced that diverticular disease was actually caused by a lack of dietary fiber. The same study showed that adding fiber to the diet cured the problem or significantly reduced the symptoms in up to 90 percent of all patients.

Wheat and Ulcers: As with diverticular disease, a bland diet has long been the treatment of choice for stomach ulcers. And just as with diverticular disease, it was the wrong approach. Ulcers develop when acids and enzymes in the stomach, which are supposed to digest food, begin "eating" the stomach lining. But fiber helps to correct the problem. In a study of 42 ulcer patients, only 14 percent of those on a high-fiber diet suffered relapses, compared to nearly 80 percent of those on a low-fiber diet. In a similar study, 80 percent of the low-fiber patients developed new ulcers, compared to only 45 percent of those on the high-fiber diet.

No one knows exactly how fiber helps to relieve and prevent ulcers. It may be that fiber helps to regulate the acids and enzymes in the stomach fluid. Perhaps the fiber toughens the lining of the stomach by mildly irritating it. Some researchers have suggested that at least some ulcers are caused by bacteria, and that wheat has antibacterial properties.

Including the Food in Your Diet

Studies at various centers around the world have produced somewhat different results, but it appears that between ¼ and ⅓ cup of wheat bran cereal per day, or several slices of whole-wheat bread, will provide the maximum health benefits. Individuals vary greatly, however, and some may require more or less.

Caution: Wheat is a common allergen (substance which causes allergies). If you feel in any way ill or "different" after eating wheat or foods containing wheat, see your doctor.

WHOLE-WHEAT FLOUR
1 cup

Calories	400
Protein	16 gm
Carbohydrate	85.2 gm
Fat	2.4 gm
Cholesterol	0 mg
Dietary Fiber	15.1 gm

	Amount	RDA
Thiamin	0.7 mg	46%
Niacin	5.2 mg	26%
Riboflavin	.1 mg	5%
Folacin	57.6 mcg	28%

 WINE

Wine has a long history of use and, unfortunately, abuse. Wine's medicinal properties are mentioned 191 times in the Bible. Ancient Jewish writings note that "Wine is the foremost of all medicines." St. Paul echoed that sentiment, writing, "... use a little wine for thine stomach's sake and thine often infirmities." The ancient Egyptians and other cultures used wine for constipation, tapeworms, coughs, and urinary problems.

Wine's Healing Properties

Although the harmful effects of alcohol are well documented, the beverage's healing effects are often overlooked. Careful study at research centers in this country and abroad have shown that moderate amounts of alcohol may help to:

- Raise HDL cholesterol
- Lower LDL cholesterol
- Reduce stress
- "Thin" the blood

Wine has also been used since ancient times as an anti-infection medicine. Studies have shown that wine kills *E. coli*, *Salmonella*, *Staphylococcus*, cholera, typhoid, and other germs.

What Scientists Have Learned About Wine

Wine and Heart Disease: A great deal of evidence shows a positive relationship between moderate alcohol intake and a reduced rate of heart disease. The findings include:

- A study of 7,705 Japanese men living in Hawaii in which the men who drank moderate amounts had less heart disease than those who drank little or no alcohol
- A drop in heart attacks among 1,505 Scottish men with high blood pressure who drank moderately
- A 1991 Harvard University study which found that drinking ½ to 1 drink per day cut the rate of heart disease by slightly over 20 percent
- In the noted Framingham study, the lowest rate of coronary heart disease was found in those who drank 1.7 to 3.4 drinks a day
- Fewer heart attacks among 11,121 Yugoslavian men ages 35 to 60 who drank daily, as compared to occasional drinkers
- A study of 1,832 white males in Chicago, which showed lower rates of cardiovascular disease in those who consumed 1 to 4 drinks per day

Moderate amounts of alcohol may benefit the heart by increasing the good cholesterol that protects against heart disease, while lowering the LDL cholesterol that harms the heart. Moderate alcohol consumption also appears to thin the blood and reduce stress.

Alcohol and the Blood: Blood clots that get stuck in an already-narrowed coronary artery can block the flow of fresh blood to the heart muscle and trigger a heart attack. In fact, studies have shown that you can predict who will have a heart attack by measuring how easily their blood platelets "stick" together to form blood clots.

In 1990, researchers reported that platelets became less likely to stick together and form clots if red wine was consumed daily for as little as two weeks. (White wine and diluted alcohol did not produce the same beneficial effect.) The anti-clotting ingredient in wine may be resveratrol, a substance which comes from grape skins.

Wine and Stress: The link between stress and heart disease is well established. So is alcohol's ability to reduce stress. As England's Dr. Thomas Stuttaford writes: "In moderate amounts, alcohol reduces anxiety, calms the emotions and thereby diminishes stress.... Alcohol diminished tension, self-consciousness and depression...."

The stress relief provided by moderate amounts of alcohol may help to reduce spasms of the coronary arteries, thus helping to keep these vital arteries open and the blood flowing.

Alcohol's effects on cholesterol, blood clotting, and stress may explain the "French Paradox." The French, who eat large amounts of fatty cheese and rich sauces, and whose cholesterols and blood pressures are as high as the average American's, have only one-third the heart disease. Many scientists believe that the French habit of drinking a glass of wine at mealtime counteracts the harmful effects of their fatty diet.

Including the Drink in Your Diet

If you already drink moderate amounts of wine, you may benefit from 1 to 2 glasses of red wine per day.

Caution: Wine has potentially serious "side effects." If you do not drink, do not start drinking in order to benefit from wine's ability to protect the heart. Instead, make other dietary changes that will confer similar benefits.

Chronic intake of high levels of alcohol may lead to elevations in blood pressure, an increased risk of heart disease, liver and brain damage, and other serious physical and social problems.

Alcohol can interfere with the body's ability to absorb calcium from food, so women who drink more than 2 glasses of wine a day may have an increased risk of osteoporosis (thinning of the bones).

Wine may also trigger headaches in sensitive individuals.

WINE, RED TABLE
3½ fluid oz

Calories	76	
Protein	.2 gm	
Carbohydrate	2.5 gm	
Fat	0 gm	
Cholesterol	0 mg	
Dietary Fiber	0 gm	

	Amount	RDA
Niacin	0.1 mg	.5%
Potassium	166 mg	NA

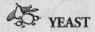 YEAST

Bread has been eaten for thousands of years, but it was only in the 1800s, thanks to the work of French scientist Louis Pasteur, that we learned why it rises when left to sit before baking. Earlier bakers knew that adding in a piece of uncooked "starter" dough saved from a previous loaf, or mixing in sediment from beer barrels would cause bread to leaven, but they didn't know why. Pasteur established that a fungus called yeast causes bread to rise by releasing gas into the dough.

Although adding yeast to dough while making bread was a widespread practice, some American health enthusiasts of the nineteenth century preferred to eat their bread unleavened. Reverend Sylvester Graham, after whom the graham cracker is named, insisted that yeast was impure and poisonous. And the designers of the Boston Water Cure, an interesting therapy of the same era, asserted that bread is "rotted by fermentation," turning health-giving bread into poison.

Yeast's Healing Properties

Yeast contains folic acid and pantothenic acid, while brewer's yeast contains biotin, chromium, and zinc. Studies published in mainstream medical journals suggest that yeast may help to:

• Relieve acne
• Reduce the risk of heart disease

What Scientists Have Learned About Yeast

Yeast and Acne: Research has suggested that the Western diet is associated with an increase in acne, and that adding yeast to the diet can help to relieve some cases of it. A 1984 study of 10 acne patients found that 2 teaspoons of high-chromium yeast daily produced rapid improvement in skin condition.

Yeast and Chromium: Yeast is one of the best sources of chromium, with 3½ ounces supplying 112 micrograms of the trace mineral. In addition to playing a role in the glucose tolerance factor (GTF), which helps to control blood sugar in diabetics, chromium guards against heart disease by protecting the linings of the arteries from being damaged by oxidation. Thanks to the large amount of refined foods and sugars in the standard American diet, marginal deficiencies of chromium are widespread. Restoring chromium to healthy levels can help people lower weight, increase their lean body mass (muscle as opposed to fat), lower cholesterol and blood fats, and improve the body's ability to regulate blood sugar.

Yeast and Heart Disease: Studies have shown that yeast supplements can protect against heart attacks by raising the HDL ("good") cholesterol while lowering the LDL ("bad") cholesterol. One yeast-heart disease study described in the *Journal of the American College of Nutrition* involved 26 healthy volunteers. After eight weeks of brewer's yeast supplements, the total cholesterol had fallen and the beneficial HDL had risen in 18 of the 26 subjects. Another study involved 24 elderly patients who were given chromium-rich brewer's yeast. After eight weeks, the average total cholesterol had fallen significantly.

Including the Food in Your Diet

Less than an ounce (20 grams) of brewer's yeast a day is enough to lower the risk of heart disease. Two teaspoons a day of high-chromium yeast may help to relieve certain cases of acne. You can purchase powdered yeast, which can be sprinkled on cereal or other foods, or mixed in shakes and juices.

> *Caution:* Those with candida, a yeast-related disorder which can cause bloating, gas, skin rashes, vaginal, and other problems, should avoid taking yeast.

YEAST, BREWER'S
1 tablespoon

	Amount	
Calories	23	
Protein	3.1 gm	
Carbohydrate	3.1 gm	
Fat	0.1 gm	
Cholesterol	0 mg	
Dietary Fiber	—	

	Amount	RDA
Riboflavin	0.3 mg	17%
Niacin	3.0 mg	15%
Thiamin	1.2 mg	8%

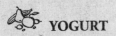 **YOGURT**

Although yogurt has been a staple food in Eastern Europe, Asia, and the Middle East for centuries, relatively few Americans consumed it until the 1970s. In fact, yogurt was not produced commercially in the United States until 1931. Fruit was first added by the Dannon company in the early 1940s to make the sour dairy food more acceptable to the American palate. (The company was named after the founder's son, Daniel.) The amount of yogurt eaten per capita increased 35 times between 1955 and 1980, and it is now a popular "health" food.

Yogurt's Healing Properties

Plain, low-fat yogurt is an excellent source of vitamin B_{12} and calcium, as well as magnesium and potassium. Studies show that yogurt may help to:

- Boost the immune system
- Ward off yeast infections
- Treat and prevent diarrhea

What Scientists Have Learned About Yogurt

Yogurt, the Immune System, and Infections: Studies at the University of California, Davis, have shown that as little as 16 ounces of yogurt (with live cultures) a day increases the levels of an immune system soldier called gamma-interferon. Yogurt also helps to fight viruses and tumors by increasing the activity of the immune system's NK (natural killer) cells.

People who regularly eat yogurt have been found to suffer from fewer colds, and to suffer less from allergies and hay fever. University of California students and senior citizens eating ¾ cup of yogurt daily had some 25 percent fewer colds during a year-long study period than their non-yogurt-eating peers.

Women who regularly eat good amounts of yogurt containing live active acidolophilus cultures are relatively free of the yeast infection called Candida albicans that plagues so many women in the Western world.

Different ingredients in yogurt also have been found to disarm carcinogens in the intestinal tract and block lung cancer in laboratory animals.

Yogurt and Diarrhea: As little as 6 ounces of yogurt a day may reduce susceptibility to diarrhea, or help relieve diarrhea that has already struck. More than 30 years ago, doctors in New York City treated infants suffering from severe diarrhea with either yogurt or a popular antidiarrheal drug. The infants given yogurt recovered twice as fast as those given the medicine.

Including the Food in Your Diet

To get the full health benefits of yogurt, add two 8-ounce servings of nonfat yogurt a day to your diet. Low-fat or nonfat yogurt is preferable. Rather than purchase yogurt with added sugary fruit sauce, slice up and add your own fresh fruit to plain yogurt.

A cup of low-fat or nonfat yogurt a day helps young bones to grow, and provides calcium to keep older bones in shape. Menopausal women should be especially careful to make sure they take in enough calcium (1500 mg per day). Premenopausal women need approximately 1000 mg of calcium per day. To make sure they get this, it is suggested that they drink either two glasses of skim milk and eat one cup of yogurt per day, or have two cups of yogurt and one glass of milk.

If the yogurt is repasteurized after the culture has been added, the crucial yogurt culture will be killed. Repasteurized yogurt is labeled "heat-treated after culturizing." "Live" or "active" yogurt has not been repasteurized, and the carton will indicate that the yogurt contains "active" or "living" cultures. "Live" culture-containing yogurt provides *probiotics,* the "good" bacteria that keep the intestines healthy. Yogurt containing live cultures is often well-tolerated by people who cannot drink milk due to a lactose intolerance.

YOGURT, PLAIN, LOW-FAT
1 cup

Calories	144	
Protein	11.9 gm	
Carbohydrate	16.0 gm	
Fat	3.5 gm	
Cholesterol	14 mg	
Dietary Fiber	0.0 gm	
	Amount	RDA
Vitamin B_{12}	1.28	64%
Calcium	415	35%
Magnesium	40	10%
Potassium	531	NA

Appendix

The Optimal Health Eating Plan

Now that you know the health-giving attributes of nearly one hundred foods, you can mix and match them to create countless delightful, tasty meals. Here are some suggestions for a week's worth of menus. These are just ideas to get you started, so feel free to adjust them to your needs and tastes, and to the availability of foods at different times of the year.

MONDAY

Breakfast
- Bagel with low-fat cream cheese
- Grapefruit
- Hot cocoa made with nonfat milk
- Orange juice

Lunch
- Salad made with water-packed tuna, tomato, shredded carrot, cucumber, lettuce, green onion, and low-fat salad dressing (optional)
- Whole-wheat roll
- Fresh fruit
- Nonfat milk

Dinner
- Stir-fried vegetables with chicken
- Brown rice
- Fruit compote
- Nonfat milk

TUESDAY

Breakfast
- Cantaloupe
- Oatmeal
- Whole-wheat toast
- Nonfat milk
- Orange juice

Lunch
- Split pea soup
- Whole-wheat toast
- Green salad made with spinach, carrots, and cabbage
- Low-fat salad dressing (optional)
- Sliced peaches
- Nonfat milk

Dinner
- Broiled salmon
- Wild rice
- Fresh green beans
- Sliced tomatoes
- Fresh fruit compote

WEDNESDAY

Breakfast
- Nonfat yogurt plus fruit of your choice, blended
- Whole-wheat toast
- Nonfat milk
- Cranberry juice

Lunch
- Pasta with stir-fried vegetables and strips of chicken breast
- Sliced oranges and bananas

- Pudding made with nonfat milk
- Nonfat milk

Dinner
- Lentil soup
- Assorted steamed vegetables
- Whole-wheat rolls
- Fresh raspberries
- Nonfat milk

THURSDAY

Breakfast
- Whole-grain cereal (hot or cold)
- Whole-wheat toast
- Orange juice
- Nonfat milk

Lunch
- Chinese chicken salad made with broiled chicken breast, bok choy, green onions, bean sprouts, and small amount of dressing (optional)
- Whole-wheat, low-fat crackers
- Papaya
- Nonfat yogurt
- Nonfat milk

Dinner
- Roast turkey (white meat only)
- Baked potato
- Steamed broccoli
- Baked squash
- Fresh fruit compote
- Nonfat milk

FRIDAY

Breakfast
- Poached egg on whole-wheat toast
- Cranberry juice
- Hot cocoa made with nonfat milk

Lunch
- Cooked red beans and rice
- Cucumber, tomato, and onion salad with low-fat dressing
- Whole-wheat bread
- Sliced banana
- Nonfat yogurt
- Nonfat milk

Dinner
- Broiled sea bass
- Pasta
- Mushrooms sautéed in low-fat margarine
- Artichoke, steamed
- Sliced nectarines
- Nonfat milk

SATURDAY

Breakfast
- Bagel spread with ricotta cheese, cinnamon, and just a dash of honey, then broiled
- Cantaloupe
- Orange juice
- Nonfat milk

Lunch
- Green pepper stuffed with ground turkey and tomato sauce
- Spinach salad with low-fat dressing
- Whole-wheat rolls
- Apricot-banana compote
- Nonfat milk

Dinner
- Linguine with clams, red peppers, and broccoli
- Steamed eggplant
- Fresh fruit salad
- Pudding made with nonfat milk

SUNDAY

Breakfast
- Whole-wheat pancakes made with low-fat margarine
- Small amounts of honey or syrup
- Berry compote
- Nonfat milk

Lunch
- Zucchini quiche made with egg substitute, nonfat milk, and low-fat cheese
- Brown rice
- Endive salad with low-fat dressing
- Sliced apple
- Nonfat milk

Dinner
- Roast chicken, white meat only
- Baked potato
- Fennel and orange salad
- Baked butternut squash
- Whole-wheat roll
- Fresh cherries

Sources

Introduction

Catherine Woteki, Director of the Food & Nutrition Board, quoted in the *New York Times,* February 19, 1992.

Position of the American Dietetic Association: phytochemicals and functional foods. *J Am Diet Assoc* Apr; 95(4):493–6, 1995.

Chapter 2

Recommended Dietary Allowances, 10th edition. Subcommittee on the 10th Edition of the RDAs, Food and Nutrition Board, Commission on Life Sciences, National Research Council. Washington, D.C.: National Academy Press, 1989.

Chapter 3

Anderson RA, Kozlovsky AS. Chromium intake, absorption and excretion of subjects consuming self-selected diets. *Am J Clin Nutr* 41:1177–83, 1985.

Armstrong PL. Iron deficiency in adolescents. *Br. Med J.* 298:499, 1989.

Costello RB, Moser-Veillon PB. A review of magnesium intake in the elderly. A cause for concern? *Magnes Res* 5(1):61–7, 1992.

Franz KB. Magnesium intake during pregnancy. Magnesium 6:18–27, 1987.

Morgan KJ, et al. Magnesium and calcium dietary intakes of the U.S. population. *J Am Coll Nutr* 4:195, 1985.

NIH· Consensus Conference: Osteoporosis. *JAMA* 252(6):799–802, 1984. Chapuy M, et al. Calcium and vitamin D supplements: Effect on calcium metabolism in elderly people. *Am J Clin Nutr* 46:324–28, 1987.

Recommended Dietary Allowances, 19th edition. Subcommittee on the 10th Edition of the RDAs, Food and Nutrition Board, Commission on Life Sciences, National Research Council. Washington, D.C.: National Academy Press, 1989.

Schoenemann HM, et al. Consequences of severe copper deficiency are independent of dietary carbohydrate in young pigs. *Am J Clin Nutr* 52:147–54, 1990.

Seelig M. *Magnesium Deficiency in the Pathogenesis of Disease.* New York: Plenum Press, 1980.

Suboptimal nutrition and behavior in children, in *Contemporary Development in Nutrition.* St. Louis, MO: CV Mosby, 1981:524–62.

Touitou Y, et al. Prevalence of magnesium and potassium deficiencies in the elderly. *Clin Chem* 33:518–23, 1987.

Wester PO. Magnesium. *Am J Clin Nutr* 45(S Suppl): 1305–12, 1987.

Chapter 5

A Consumer's Guide to Medicines In Food. Ruth Winter. New York: Crown Trade Paperbacks, 1995.

Abbasi AA, et al. Experimental zinc deficiency in man: Effect on testicular function. *J Lab Clin Med* 96(3):554–50, 1980.

Al-Nakib W, et al. Prophylaxis and treatment of rhinovirus colds with zinc gluconate lozenges. *J Antimicrob Chemother* 20(6):893–901, 1987.

Alexander M, et al. Oral beta-carotene can increase the number of OKT4+ cells in human blood. *Immunol Lett* 9:221–24, 1985.

Anderson JW, Tietyen-Clark J. Dietary fiber: Hyperlipidemia, hypertension, and coronary heart disease. *Am J Gastroenterol* 81(10): 907–19, 1986.

Anderson RA, Kozlovsky AS. Chromium intake, absorption and excretion of subjects consuming self-selected diets. *Am J Clin Nutr* 41:1177–83, 1985.

Apitz-Castro R; Badimon JJ; Badimon L. A garlic derivative, ajoene, inhibits platelet deposition on severely damaged vessel wall in an in vivo porcine experimental model. *Thromb Res* Aug 1;75(3):243–9, 1994.

Armstrong PL. Iron deficiency in adolescents. *Br Jed J.* 298:499, 1989.

Bach R, et al. Effects of fish oil capsules in two dosages on blood pressure, platelet functions, haemorheological and clinical chemistry parameters in apparently healthy subjects. *Ann Nutr Metab* 33:359–67, 1989.

Baig MM, Cerda JJ. Pectin: Its interaction with serum lipoproteins. *Am J Clin Nutr* 34:50–53, 1981.

Baly D, et al. Effect of manganese deficiency on insulin binding, glucose transport and metabolism in rat adipocytes. *J Nutr* 120: 1075–9, 1990.

Baum G, et al. Meclozine and pyridoxine in pregnancy. *Practitioner* 190:251, 1963.

Bendich A. Carotenoids and the immune system. *J Nutr* 119:112–115, 1989.

Berge K, Canner P. Coronary Drug Project; Experience with niacin. *Eur J Clin Pharmacol* 40:S49–51, 1991.

Bergmann KE, et al. Abnormalities of hair zinc concentration in mothers of newborn infants with spina bifida. *Am J Clin Nutr* 33: 2145, 1980.

Bernat I, Iron deficiency, in *Iron Metabolism.* New York, Plenum Press, 1983:215–74.

Bhathema S, et al. Decreased plasma enkephalins in copper deficiency in man. *Am J Clin Nutr* 43:42–46, 1986.

Bjorneboe A, et al. Effect of dietary supplementation with eicosapentaenoic acid in the treatment of atopic dermatitis. *Br J Dermatol* 117(4):463–69, 1987.

Block G. Epidemiologic evidence regarding vitamin C and cancer. *Am J Clin Nutr* 54:1310S–14S, 1991.

Blondell JM. The anticarcinogenic effect of magnesium. *Med Hypotheses* 6:863–871, 1980.

Blood S, Peric-Golia L. Myocardial calcification, acute infarction, and Mg in drinking water: Salt Lake City vs Washington DC. Abstract. *J Am Coll Nutr* 8(5):455, 1989.

Blue Corn & Square Tomatoes. Rebecca Rupp. Pownal, VT: Garden Way Publishing, 1987.

Bond GG, et al. Dietary vitamin A and lung cancer: Results of a case-control study among chemical workers. *Nutr Cancer* 9:109–21, 1987.

Borgman RF, Dietary factors in essential hypertension. *Prog Food Nutr Sci* 9:109–47, 1985.

Botez, MI, et al. Neuropsychological correlates of folic acid deficiency: facts and hypotheses. In Boetz MI, Reynolds EH, eds. *Folic Acid in Neurology, Psychiatry, and Internal Medicine.* New York: Raven Press, 435–61, 1979.

Brown RR, et al. Correlation of serum retinol levels with response to chemotherapy in breast cancer. Meeting Abstract. *Proc Am Assoc Cancer Res* 22:184, 1981.

Buamah PK, et al. Maternal zinc status: A determinant of central nervous system malformation. *Br J Obstet Gynaecol* 91:788–90, 1984.

Buch IM, et al. Presentation on Zinc and the prostate. Presented at the annual meeting of the Am Med Assoc, Chicago, 1974.

Buetler E, et al. Iron therapy in chronically fatigued non-anemic women: A double blind study. *Ann Intern Med* 52:378, 1960.

Burch GE, Giles TD. The importance of magnesium deficiency in cardiovascular diseases. *Am Heart J* 94:649–57, 1977.

Burr ML, et al. Effects of changes in fat, fish and fibre intakes on death and myocardial reinfarction: diet and reinfarction trial (DART). *Lancet* 2:757–61, 1989.

Butterworth CE, et al. Improvement in cervical dysplasia associated with folic acid therapy in users of oral contraceptives. *Am J Clin Nutr* 35(1):73–82, 1982.

Calvert RJ, et al. *J Natl Cancer Inst* 79(4):875, 1987. Steineck G, et al. Vitamin A supplements, fried foods, fat and urothelial cancer. A case-referent study in Stockholm in 1985–87. *Int J Cancer* 45:1006–11, 1990.

Caroll KK. Dietary fats and cancer. *Am J Clin Nutr* 53:1064S–7S, 1991.

Carslaw RW, Neill J. Vitamin B_{12} is psorasis. Letter. *Br Med J* 1:611, 1963.

Cathcart RF. Glutathione and HIV infection. Letter. *Lancet* 1:235, 1990.

Cathcart RF. Vitamin C in the treatment of acquired immune deficiency syndrome (AIDS). *Med Hypotheses* 14(4):423–33, 1984.

Cerda JC, et al. The effect of grapefruit pectin on patients at risk for coronary heart disease without altering diet or lifestyle. *Clin Cardiol* 11(9):589–94, 1988.

Chapuy M, et al. Calcium and vitamin D supplements: Effect on calcium metabolism in elderly people. *Am J Clin Nutr* 46:324–28, 1987.

Cheraskin E, et al. Daily vitamin C consumption and fatigability. *J Am Geriatr Soc* 24(3):136–37, 1976.

Cloarec MJ, et al. Alpha-tocopherol: Effect on plasma lipoproteins in hypercholesterolemic patients. *Isr J Med Sci* 32(8):869–72, 1987.

Collip PJ, et al. Pyridoxine treatment of childhood bronchial asthma. *Ann Allergy* 35:93–7, 1975.

Creter D, et al. Effect of vitamin E on platelet aggregation in diabetic retinopathy. *Acta Hematol* 62:74, 1979.

Criqui MH, et al. Dietary alcohol, calcium and potassium. Independent and combined effects on blood pressure. *Circulation* 80(3):609–14, 1989.

Davidson MH. Fish oils vs. total lipid profile. Letter. *Med World News* Feb 22, p. 10, 1988.

Davis WH, et al. Monotherapy with magnesium increases abnormally high density lipoprotein cholesterol: A clinical essay. *Curr Ther Res* 36:341, 1984.

de Fabio A. Treatment & prevention of osteoarthritis. *Townsend Letter for Doctors.* February–March 143–48, 1990.

de Vries N, Snow GB. Relationships of vitamins A and E and beta-carotene serum levels to head and neck cancer patients with and without second primary tumors. *Eur Arch Otorhinolaryngol* 247: 368–70, 1990.

Dychner T, Wester PO. Magnesium and potassium in serum and muscle in relation to disturbances of cardiac rhythm. In: *Magnesium in Health and Disease.* Spectrum Publishing Company, pp. 551–7, 1980.

Dyer A, Stamler J, Berkson P, Leper M, McKean H, Shekeele R, Lindbert H, Garside D. Alcohol consumption, cardiovascular risk factors and mortality in two Chicago epidemiological studies. *Circulation* 56, 1977.

Earl Mindell. *Earl Mindell's Food as Medicine.* New York: Fireside Books, 1994.

Elsborg L, et al. The intake of vitamin and minerals by the elderly at home. *Int J Vitamin Nutr Res* 53:321–29, 1983.

Elwood JC, et al. Effect of high-chromium brewer's yeast on human serum lipids. *J Am Coll Nutr* I:263–74, 1982.

Ernst E, et al. Garlic and blood lipids. *Br Med J* 291:139, 1985.

Esk C, et al. Correlation of plasma ascorbic acid with cardiovascular risk factors. *Clin Res* 38:A747, 1990.

Fahim MS, et al. Zinc treatment for the reduction of hyperplasia of the prostate. *Fed Proc* 35:361, 1976. Presentation by Buch IM, et al. Zinc and the prostate. Presented at the annual meeting of the Am Med Assoc, Chicago, 1974.

Finch CA. Editorial: Evaluation of iron status. *JAMA* 251(15):2004, 1984.

Finehart JF, Greenberg LD. Arteriosclerotic lesions in pyridoxine deficient monkeys. *Am J Pathol* 25:481–96, 1949.

Fontham ETH, et al. Dietary vitamins A and C and lung cancer risk in Louisiana. *Cancer* 62:2267–73, 1988.

Franz KB. Magnesium intake during pregnancy. *Magnesium* 6:18–27, 1987.

Fraser GE, et al. A possible protective effect of nut consumption on risk of coronary heart disease. *Arch Int Med* 152:1416–24, 1992.

Friday KE, et al. Omega-3 fatty acid supplementation has discordant effects on plasma glucose and lipoproteins in type II diabetes. Abstract. *Diabetes* 36(Suppl 1):12A, 1987.

Gaziano JM. Harvard U. Presentation at the Am Heart Assoc Scientific Session, Dallas. Reported in *Med World News,* January 1991.

Gey KF, et al. Inverse correlation between plasma vitamin E and mortality from ischemic heart disease in cross-cultural epidemiology. *Am J Clin Nutr* 53:326S–34S, 1991.

Ginter E, et al. Vitamin C in the control of hypercholesterolemia in man. *Int J Vitamin Nutr Res* Suppl 23:137–52, 1982.

Glauber H, et al. Adverse metabolic effect of omega-3 fatty acids in non-insulin dependent diabetes mellitus. *Ann Intern Med* 108(5): 663–68, 1988.

Glueck CK, et al. Amelioration of severe migraine with omega-3 fatty acids. A double-blind, placebo-controlled clinical trial. Abstract. *Am J Clin Nutr* 43:710, 1986.

Goldberg J, et al. Factors associated with age-related macular degeneration. An analysis of data from the first National Health and Nutrition Examination Survey. *Am J Epidemiol* 128(4):700–10, 1988.

Graham S, et al. Dietary factors in the epidemiology of cancer of the larynx. *Am J Epidemiol* 113(6):675–80, 1981.

Griffith RS, et al. Success of L-lysine therapy in frequently recurrent herpes simplex infection. *Dermatologica* 175:183–90, 1987.

Guo W, et al. Correlations of dietary intake and blood nutrient levels with oesphageal cancer mortality in China. *Nutr Cancer* 13:121–27, 1990.

Gupta S. Effect of radiotherapy on plasma ascorbic acid concentration in cancer patients. Unpublished thesis summarized in Hanck AB, Vitamin C and Cancer. *Prog Clin Biol Res* 259:307–20, 1988.

Haglund O, et al. The effects of fish oil on triglycerides, cholesterol, fibrinogen, and malondialdehyde in humans supplemented with vitamin E. *J Nutr* 121:165–9, 1991.

Hallfrisch J, et al. High plasma vitamin C associated with increased plasma HDL-and HDL2-cholesterol. *Clin Res* 39A203, 1991.

Harlan WE, et al. Blood pressure and nutrition in adults. The National Health and Nutrition Examination Survey. *Am J Epidemiol* 120: 17–27, 1984.

Harris RC, et al. A case-control study of dietary carotene in men with lung cancer and in men with epithelial cancer. *Nutr Cancer* 15: 63–8, 1991.

Heinle H, Betz E. Effects of dietary garlic supplementation in a rat model of atherosclerosis. *Arzneimittelforschung* May; 44(5):614–7, 1994.

Hendra T, et al. Effects of fish oil supplements in NIDDM subjects. *Diab Care* 13:821–29, 1990.

Higashi A, et al. A prospective survey of serial serum zinc levels and pregnancy outcome. *J Ped Gastroenterol* 7:430–33, 1988.

Hirose N, et al. Inhibition of cholesterol absorption and synthesis in rats by sesamin. *J Lipid Research* 32:629–38, 1991.

Hoagland PD, Pferrer PE. *J Agric Food Chem* May/June, 1987.

Holland OB, et al. Ventricular ectopic activity with diuretic therapy. *Am J Hypertens* 1(4 Pt 1):380–85, 1988.

Howe G, et al. Dietary factors and risk of breast cancer: Combined analysis of 12 case-control studies. *J Natl Cancer Inst* 82:561–9, 1990.

Hsing A, et al. Serologic precursors of cancer: retinol, carotenoids, tocopherol and risk of prostate cancer. *J Natl Cancer Inst* 82:941–46, 1990.

Immune for Life. Arnold Fox and Barry Fox. Rocklin, CA: Prima Publishing, 1989.

Ip C, Lisk DJ. Enrichment of selenium in allium vegetables for cancer prevention. *Carcinogenesis* Sep;15(9):1881–5, 1994.

Joeg JM, et al. special communication.: An approach to the management of hyperlipoproteinemia. *JAMA* 25(4):512–21, 1986.

Johnson, P. Human Nutrition Center, US Dept. of Agriculture. Reported in *Townsend Letter for Doctors,* May, 1991.

Judge TG, Cowan NR. Dietary potassium intake and grip strength in older people. *Gerontologia clinica* 13:221–26, 1971.

Kafka H, et al. Serum magnesium and potassium in acute myocardial infarction. Influence on ventricular arrhythmias. *Arch Intern Med* 147(3):465–69. 1987.

Kaizer L, et al. Fish consumption and breast cancer risk: An ecological study. *Nutr Cancer* 12:61–68, 1989.

Kaul L, et al. The role of diet in prostate cancer. *Nutr Cancer* 9:123–28, 1987.

Keenan J, et al. Niacin revisited: A randomized, controlled trial of wax-matrix sustained-release niacin in hypercholesterolemia. *Arch Intern Med* 151:1424–32, 1991.

Khaw KT, Barrett-Connor E. Dietary potassium and stroke-associated mortality. A 12-year prospective population study. *N Engl J Med* 316(5):235–40, 1987.

Kline G. Reported in *Med World News,* 4/24/89.

Knekt P, et al. Serum vitamin A and subsequent risk of cancer: Cancer incidence follow-up of the Finnish Mobile Clinic Health Examination Survey. *Am J Epidemiol* 132:857–70, 1990.

Knekt P, et al. Vitamin E and cancer prevention. *Am J Clin Nutr* 53: 283S–6S, 1991.

Kolonel LN, et al. Vitamin A and prostate cancer in elderly men:

Enhancement of risk. *Cancer Res* 47(11):2982–85, 1987.

Kozarevic D, Vojvadie N, Kaelber C, Gordon T, McGee D, Zukel W. Drinking habits and death: The Yugoslavian cardiovascular disease study. *Int'l J Epidemiol* 12, 1983.

Krinksy NI. Effect of carotenoids in cellular and animal systems. *Am J Clin Nutr* 53:238S–46S, 1991.

Kromhout D, et al. The inverse relation between fish consumption and 20-year mortality from coronary heart disease. *N Engl J Med* 312:1205–9, 1985.

Kromhout D. n-3 fatty acids and coronary heart disease. *B N F Nutr Bull* 15:93–102, 1990.

Kune GA, et al. Serum levels of beta-carotene, vitamin A and zinc in male lung cancer cases and controls. *Nutr Cancer* 12:169–76, 1989.

Kune S, et al. Case-control study of dietary etiological factors: the Melbourne Colorectal Cancer Study. *Nutr Cancer* 9:21–42, 1987.

Kushi LH, et al. Diet and 20-mortality from coronary heart disease. The Ireland-Boston Diet-Herat Study. *N Engl J Med* 312(13):811–18, 1985.

Kyrtopoulos SA. Ascorbic acid and the formation of N-nitroso compounds: possible role of ascorbic acid in cancer prevention. *Am J Clin Nutr* 45:1344–50, 1987.

Lane BC, Diet and the glaucomas. Abstract. *J Am Coll Nutr* 19(5): 536, 1991.

Lane BC. Evaluation of intraocular pressure with daily, sustained closework stimulus to accommodation, lowered tissue, chromium and dietary deficiency of ascorbic acid. 3rd Intl Conf. on Myopia, Copenhagen & The Hague. *Doc Ophthalmol* 28:149–55, 1981.

Lazebnik N, et al. Zinc status, pregnancy complications, and labor abnormalities. *Am J Obstet Gynecol* 158(10):161–66, 1988.

LeGardeur BY, et al. A case-controlled study of serum vitamin A, E and C in lung cancer patients. *Nutr Cancer* 14:133–40, 1990.

Leonard PJ, Losowsky MS. Effect of alpha-tocopherol administration on red cell survival in vitamin E-deficient human subjects. *Am J Clin Nutr* 24:388–93, 1971.

Linner E. The pressure lowering effect of ascorbic acid in ocular hypertension. *Acta Ophthalmol* (Copen) 47:685–9, 1969.

Lipman T, et al. Esophageal zinc content in human squamous esophageal cancer. *J Am Coll Nutr* 6:41–46, 1987.

Lubotz, WC. The structure and function of the sebaceous glands. *Arch Dermatol* 76:162–71, 1957.

Luria MH. Effect of low-dose niacin on high-density lipoprotein cholesterol and total cholesterol/high density lipoprotein cholesterol ratio. *Arch Intern Med* 148:2493–95, 1988.

Magnesium Deficiency in the Pathogenesis of Disease. M. Selig. New York: Plenum Press, 1980.

Malhotra A, et al. Placental zinc in normal and intra-uterine growth-retarded pregnancies. *Br J Nutr* 63:613–21, 1990.

Martin N; Bardisa L; Pantoja C; Vargas M; and others. Anti-arrhythmic profile of a garlic dialysate assayed in dogs and isolated atrial preparations. *J Ethnopharmacol* Jun; 43(1):1–8, 1994.

McCarren T, et al. Amelioration of severe migraine by fish oil (w-3) fatty acids. Abstract. *Am J Clin Nutr* 41:874a, 1985.

McCarron DA, et al. Blood pressure and nutrient intake in the United States. *Science* 224(4656):1392–98, 1984.

McCarron DA, et al. Dietary calcium and blood pressure: modifying factors in specific populations. *Am J Clin Nutr* 54:215S–19S, 1991.

Mensiunk R, et al. Effects of monounsaturated fatty acids versus complex carbohydrates on serum lipoproteins and apoproteins in healthy men and women. *Metabolism* 38:172–78, 1989.

Messina M, Barnes S. The role of soy products in reducing risk of cancer. *J Natl Cancer Inst* 83:541–6, 1991.

Mian E, et al. Anthocyanosides and the walls of microvessels: further aspects of the mechanism of action of their protective effect in syndromes due to abnormal capillary fragility. *Minerva Med* 68(52):3565–81, 1977.

Michalek AM, et al. Vitamin A and tumor recurrence in bladder cancer. *Cancer* 9:143–46, 1987.

Morgan KJ, et al. Magnesium and calcium dietary intakes of the U.S. population. *J Am Coll Nutr* 4:195, 1985.

Mukherjee MD, et al. Maternal zinc, iron, folic acid, protein nutriture and outcome of human pregnancy. *Am J Clin Nutr* 40(3):496–507, 1984.

Murphy SP, et al. Vitamin E intakes and sources in the United States. *Am J Clin Nutr* 52:361–67, 1990.

Nahata MC, et al. Effect of chlorophyllin on urinary odor in incontinent geriatric patients. *Drug Intelligence and Clin Pharm* 17:732–34, 1983.

Natta CL. Painful crises due to sickle-cell anemia: Effect of vitamin B$_6$ supplementation. *IM* 7(10):132–40, 1986.

Natural Alternatives to Over-the-Counter and Prescription Drugs. Michael Murray. New York: William Morrow, 1994.

Naylor GJ, et al. A double-blind placebo-controlled trial of ascorbic acid in obesity. *Nutr Health* 4:25–8, 1985.

Newsome D, et al. The trace element and antioxidant economy of the human macula: can dietary supplementation influence the course of macular degeneration? Abstract. *J Am Coll Nutr* 10(5):536, 1991.

Newsome D, et al. Oral zinc in macular degeneration. *Arch Ophthalmol* 106(2):192–8, 1988.

Newton HM, et al. The causes and correction of low blood vitamin C concentration in the elderly. *Am J Clin Nutr* 42(4):656–59, 1985.

Nielsen FH, et al. Effect of dietary boron on mineral, estrogen, and testosterone metabolism in postmenopausal women. *Fed Am Soc Exp Biol* 1(5):394–97. 1987.

NIH Consensus conference: Osteoporosis. *JAMA* 252(6):799–802, 1984.

Nordrehaug J, et al. Serum potassium concentration as a risk factor of ventricular arrhythmias early in acute myocardial infarction. *Circulation* 71(4):645–9, 1985.

Norell Se, et al. Fish consumption and mortality from coronary heart disease. *Br Med J* 293:426, 1986.

Norie IH, Foster HD. Water quality and cancer of the digestive tract: The Canadian experience. *J Orthomol Med* 4(2):59–69, 1989.

Nutritional Influences on Illness. 2nd ed. Melvin Werback. Tarzana, CA: Third Line Press, 1993.

Offenbacker Eg, Pi-Sunyer FX. Beneficial effect of chromium-rich yeast on glucose tolerance and blood lipids in elderly subjects. *Diabetes* 29:919–25, 1980.

Orr, JW, et al. Nutritional status of patients with untreated cervical cancer. II. Vitamin Assessment. *Am J Obstet Gynecol* 151(5):632–35, 1985.

Palan PR, et al. Plasma levels of antioxidant beta-carotene and alpha-tocopherol in uterine cervix dysplasias and cancer. *Nutr Cancer* 15:13–20, 1991.

Pikkar NA, Wedel M, van der Beek E, et al. Effects of moderate alcohol consumption on platelet aggregation, fibrinolysis, and blood lipids. *Metabolism* 36:538–47, 1987.

Poynard T, et al. Reduction of post-prandial insulin needs by pectin as assessed by the artificial pancreas in insulin-dependent diabetics. *Diabetes Metab* 8(3):187–89, 1982.

Prasad KN. Modulation of the effects of tumor therapeutic agents by vitamin C. *Life Sci* 27(4):275–80, 1980.

Prichard GA, et al. Lipids in breast cancinogenesis. *Br J Surg* 76(10): 10690–83, 1989.

Raloff J. Reasons for boning up on manganese. *Sci News* Sept 27: 199, 1986.

Recommended Dietary Allowances 19th edition. Subcommittee on the 10th Edition of the RDAs, Food and Nutrition Board, Commission on Life Sciences, National Research Council. Washington, D.C.: National Academy Press, 1989. p. 266.

Reich R, et al. Eicosapentaenoic acid reduces the invasive and metastatic activities of malignant tumor cells. *Biochem Biophys Res Commun* 160:559–64, 1989.

Reichman M, et al. Serum vitamin A and subsequent development of prostate cancer in the first National Health and Nutrition Examination Survey Epidemiologic Follow-up Study. *Cancer Res* 50: 2311–15, 1990.

Reuler JB, et al. Adult scurvy. *JAMA* 253(6):805–7, 1985.

Riemersma RA, et al. Risk of angina pectoris and plasma concentrations of vitamins A, C and E and carotene. *Lancet* 337:1–5, 1991.

Rinehart JF, Greenberg LD. Vitamin B₆ deficiency in the Rhesus monkey. *Am J Clin Nutr* 4:318–25, 1956.

Robbins RC, et al. Ingestion of grapefruit lowers elevated hematocrits in human subjects. *Int'l J Vitamin Nutrition Res* 58:414–17, 1988.

Rosenberg EW, Kirk BS. Acne diet reconsidered. *Arch Dermatol* 117:193–95, 1981.

Rubin D., reported in McCarty, M. High chromium yeast for acne? *Med Hypotheses* 14:307–10, 1984.

Rylander R, Bonevic H, Rubenowitz E. Magnesium and calcium in drinking water and cardiovascular mortality. *Scand J Work Environ Health* 17:91–4, 1991.

Sable-Amplis R, et al. Further studies on the cholesterol-lowering effect of apple in humans. *Nutr Res* 3:325–8, 1983.

Sahakian V, et al. Vitamin B₆ is effective therapy for nausea and vomiting of pregnancy. A randomized double-blind placebo-controlled study. *Obstet Gynecol* 78:33–36, 1991.

Sakaguchi M, et al. Relationship of tissue and tumor fatty acids to dietary fat in experimental colorectal cancer. *Gut* 30:1449, 1989.

Salamon P, et al. Treatment of ulcerative colitis with fish oil in n-3-omega fatty acid: an open trial. *J Clin Gastroenterol* 12(2):157–61, 1990.

Salonen JT, et al. Blood pressure, dietary fats, and antioxidants. *Am J Clin Nutr* 48:1226–32, 1988.

Sangiori GB, et al. Serum potassium levels, red-blood-cell potassium and alterations of the repolarization phase of electrocardiography in old subjects. *Age Ageing* 13:309, 1984.

Schoenemann HM, et al. Consequences of severe copper deficiency are independent of dietary carbohydrate in young pigs. *Am J Clin Nutr* 52:147–54, 1990.

Schwartz J, Weiss ST, Dietary factors and their relation to respiratory symptoms. The Second National Health and Nutrition Examination Survey. *Am J Epidemiol* 132(1):67–76, 1990.

Seigneur M, Bonnet J, Dorian B, et al. Effect of the consumption of alcohol, white wine and red wine on platelet function and serum lipids. *J Applied Cardiol* 5:215–22, 1990.

Silagy CA, Neil HA. A meta-analysis of the effect of garlic on blood pressure. *J Hypertens* Apr;12(4):463–8, 1994.

Singer P. Blood pressure-lowering effect of omega-3 polyunsaturated fatty acids in clinical studies. In AP Simopoulos, et al, eds. Health Effects of Omega-3 Polyunsaturated Fatty Acids in Seafoods. *World Rev Nutr Diet* 66:329–48, 1991.

Singh VN, Gaby SK. Premalignant lesions: role of antioxidant vitamins and beta-carotene in risk reduction and prevention of malignant transformation. *Am J Clin Nutr* 53:386S–90S, 1991.

Smialowicz RJ, et al. Manganese chloride enhances natural cell-mediated immune effector cell function: Effects on macrophages. *Immunopharmacol* 9:1–11, 1985.

Somer Elizabeth. *The Essential Guide to Vitamins and Minerals.* New York: HarperPerennial, 1992.

Sorenson RJ, et al. Antineoplastic activities of some copper salicylates. In DD Hemphill (ed). *Trace Substances in Environmental Health* XVI. Columbia, MO: University of Missouri, 1982.

Stahelin HB, et al. Cancers, vitamins, and plasma lipids: Prospective Basel Study. *J Natl Cancer Inst* 73(6):1463–8, 1984.

Stammers T, et al. Fish oil in osteoarthritis. Letter. *Lancet* 2:503, 1989.

Steineck G, et al. Vitamin A supplements, fried foods, fat and urothelial cancer. A case-referent study in Stockholm in 1985–87. *Int J Cancer* 45:1006–11, 1990.

Steiner M. Influence of vitamin E on platelet function in humans. *J Am Coll Nutr* 10(5):466–73, 1991.

Stich HF, et al. Use of the micronucleus test to monitor the effect of vitamin A, beta-carotene and canthaxanthin on the buccal mucosa of betel nut/tobacco chewers. *Int J Cancer* 344(6):745–50.

Stoskman JA, Iron deficiency anemia: Have we come far enough? *JAMA* 258:1645–47, 1987.

Strain JJ. A reassessment of diet and osteoporosis: Possible role for copper. *Med Hypothesis* 27(4):333–38, 1988.

Stryker W, et al. Diet, plasma levels of beta carotene and alpha tocopherol, and risk of malignant melanoma. *Am J Epidemiol* 13:597–611, 1990.

Svendsen L, Rattan SI, Clark BF. Testing garlic for possible anti-ageing effects on long-term growth characteristics, morphology and macromolecular synthesis of human fibroblasts in culture. *J Ethnopharmacol* Jul 8;43(2):125–33, 1994.

Taylor TV, et al. Ascorbic acid supplementation in the treatment of pressure-sores. *Lancet* 2:544–46, 1974.

Terahara N; Yamaguchi M; Honda T. Malonylated anthocyanins from bulbs of red onion, Allium cepa L. *Biosci Biotechnol Biochem* Jul; 58(7):1324–5, 1994.

Thaulow E, Erikssen J, Sandvic L, et al. Blood platelet count and function are related to total cardiovascular death in apparently healthy men. *Circulation* 1991;84:613–17; Trip et al., 1990.

Tikkiwal M, et al. Effect of zinc administration on seminal zinc and fertility of oligospermic males. *Indian J Physiol Pharmacol* 31(1): 30–34, 1987.

Torok B; Belagyi J; Rietz B; Jacob R. Effectiveness of garlic on the radical activity in radical generating systems. *Arzneimittelforschung* May;44(5):608–11, 1994.

Touitou Y, et al. Prevalence of magnesium and potassium deficiencies in the elderly. *Clin Chem* 33:518–23, 1987.

Travers RL, et al. Boron and arthritis: the results of a double-blind pilot study. *J Nutr Med* 1:127–32, 1990.

Travers RL, Rennie GC. Clinical trial—boron and arthritis. The results of a double blind pilot study. *Townsend Letter for Doctors*. June 1990, pp. 360–62.

Trout DL. Vitamin C and cardiovascular risk factors. *Am J Clin Nutr* 53:322S–5S, 1991.

Underwood EJ. *Trace Elements in Humans and Animal Nutrition*. 4th ed. London: Academic Press, 1977, p. 198.

Van Horn L. Serum lipid response to a fat-modified, oatmeal-enhanced diet. *Prev Med* 17(3):1988.

Verreault R, et al. A case-control study of diet and invasive cervical cancer. *Int J Cancer* 43:1050–54, 1989.

Virno M, et al. Oral treatment of glaucoma with vitamin C. *Eye, Ear, Nose, Throat Monthly*. 46:1502–8, 1967.

Wald NJ, et al. Plasma retinol, beta-carotene and vitamin E levels in relation to the future risk of breast cancer. *Br J Cancer* 49:321–4, 1984.

Wallenburg HCS, et al. Effect of oral iron supplementation during pregnancy on material and fetal iron status. *J Perinat Med* 12(1): 7–12, 1984.

Ward NI, et al. Elemental factors in human fetal development. *J Nutr Med* 1:19–26, 1990.

Welch C; Wuarin L; Sidell N. Antiproliferative effect of the garlic compound S-allyl cysteine on human neuroblastoma cells in vitro. *Cancer Lett* Apr 30;63(3):211–9, 1992.

Wester PO. Magnesium. *Am J Clin Nutr* 45(S Suppl):1305–12, 1987.

Whittemore A, et al. Diet, physical activity, and colorectal cancer among Chinese in North America and China. *J Natl Cancer Inst* 82:915–26, 1990.

Willett WC, et al. Relation of meat, fat, and fiber intake to the risk of colon cancer in a prospective study among women. *N Engl J Med* 323:1664–72, 1990.